Adolescent Pregnancy

Policy and Prevention Services, Second Edition

Naomi B. Farber, PhD, MSW, ACSW, is a member of the faculty of the College of Social Work at the University of South Carolina.

She teaches in the areas of advanced direct theory and practice. Her research has focused on adolescent sexuality and parenting, poverty and family formation, and HIV/AIDS prevention among high-risk youth.

Adolescent Pregnancy

Policy and Prevention Services, Second Edition

Naomi B. Farber, PhD, MSW, ACSW

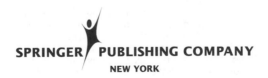

SPRINGER PUBLISHING COMPANY

NEW YORK

Springer Publishing Company, LLC
11 West 42nd Street
New York, NY 10036
www.springerpub.com

Acquisitions Editor: Jennifer Perillo
Cover Design: TG Design
Composition: Six Red Marbles

Ebook ISBN: 978-0-8261-2549-1

09 10 11 / 5 4 3 2 1

Library of Congress Cataloging-in-Publication Data

Farber, Naomi.
    Adolescent pregnancy: policy and prevention services/Naomi B. Farber.—2nd ed.
        p. cm.
    Includes bibliographical references.
    ISBN 978-0-8261-2548-4
    1. Teenage pregnancy—Government policy—United States.
    2. Teenage pregnancy—United States—Prevention. I. Title.
        HQ766.8.F37 2009
        306.874'3—dc22

                                                        2009018692

Printed in the United States of America by Hamilton

To the memory of my mother,
Ruth Diamond Farber,
and the present blessing of Steven Grosby

Contents

Contributors

Janet Shapiro, PhD
Associate Professor
Bryn Mawr College
Bryn Mawr, PA

Nancy Brown, PhD
Associate Professor
University of South Carolina
College of Social Work
Columbia, SC

Preface

In light of the continued decline in pregnancy and childbearing among adolescents in the United States subsequent to the first edition of this book, what is the need for a new edition at this time? Have we not obviated the need to revisit what apparently has been a successful effort across public and private sectors, communities, programs, and policies to address teen pregnancy? What more, or different, is there to say about teen pregnancy prevention?

There has been success in reducing rates of pregnancy and childbearing across most demographic categories of teens. This success is notable among even high-risk teens such as low-income African American youth. Although it is difficult to know which factors account for precisely how much of the widespread decline, there are some obvious, if tentative, answers. Some of the decline is attributable to medical advances in contraception; some to changes in behavior of adolescents in response to various forces in their social and cultural environments. It is certain, however, that many factors exert influence on the complex behaviors leading to early pregnancy and parenthood and have contributed to the positive trends between 1991 and 2005.

First, many pregnancies among teenagers are being prevented by effective contraception. Over time, sexually active teenagers have increased their regular use of birth control. In addition, the advent and availability of long-lasting methods of contraception that do not depend on planned use at each time of sexual intercourse or skills to use them contribute to contraceptive success. Second, there appears to be some rising conservatism in sexual activity among some teens. Studies of large, nationally representative surveys find that the age at which adolescents, both boys and girls, begin to have sex has risen slightly and that boys are reporting engaging in less sexual activity. Delaying the age of sexual initiation and fewer occasions of intercourse that might be unprotected, of course, reduce the overall risk for conceiving as a teenager outside of marriage.

It is reasonable to assume that some of the reasons for these positive changes in sexual behavior are found in the proliferation of prevention programs across the country and in the vigorous campaigns to raise public awareness mounted by local school districts, communities, states, and national organizations that are supported by public policies and private foundations. Other sources of influence are found in some communities' religious presence and families' values. It is also reasonable to assume that no single factor was responsible for the recent decline. Rather, many changes converged to create more caution among some young people when they made choices about their sexual development and behavior.

These successes, however, should not lead us to complacency about the current risks that young people, and those who have not yet reached adolescence, face regarding their sexual choices. There are several reasons for continued, and even heightened, vigilance in our attention to high-risk sexual behavior among teenagers.

Most noteworthy at present is the reversal of the decline in adolescent fertility evident during the past two years of available data. The most recent data show a small increase in 2006. The National Campaign to Prevent Teen and Unplanned Pregnancy examined this disappointing news:

> New data for 2006 from the National Center for Health Statistics indicate that the 14-year decline in the U.S. teen birthrate has reversed, and both the number of births to teens and the teen birthrate have risen. Between 2005 and 2006, the teen birthrate rose 3%, from 40.5 to 41.9 births per 1,000 females aged 15–19. The number of births to teens also rose by 20,834, from 414,593 to 435,427. *(2008, p. 1)*

In fact, this reversal was foreshadowed in the past few years by a slowing of the steep decline in fertility and a slight decrease in young women's use of birth control. In other words, prior to this shift upward in teen births, there was a plateau in the progress of the previous several years. At this time, we do not know if the latest upswing in adolescent fertility represents a trend backward, or is an anomaly that will be corrected in near future.

Even while adolescent fertility was dropping, the incidence of pregnancy and childbearing among American teens remained and continues to be far greater than other Western and industrial societies. Although economic downturns, such as has occurred recently worldwide, tend to be associated with increases in teenage pregnancy in other countries such as in the United States, the differences in rates of pregnancy between American and European, Canadian and Asian adolescents remain considerable. That is, in spite of an absolute decrease in the proportion of teens who bear children, our relative success in reducing teen pregnancy is modest.

In the context of overall and group-specific declines of pregnancy and childbearing, minority teens from low-income families continue to have first and additional children at significantly higher rates than other teens; and these disadvantaged teens are more likely to have closely spaced additional births. As the population of Hispanics in the United States increases, absolute numbers of pregnancies as well as rates of pregnancy among disadvantaged Hispanic youth remain at worrisome levels. Although fertility fell among black youth, their rates of sexually transmitted infections continue to be very high, and young black men account for a significant proportion of new cases of HIV.

The fact remains that many young people put their physical and emotional health at risk by having unprotected sex. When these risks result in pregnancy and parenthood, as they typically do among the most vulnerable youth, the consequences are, in some respects, more negative than in the past. The recent group of studies in Hoffman and Maynard's "Kids Having Kids" (2008) estimate the relative contemporary costs of a teen having a child. They find the following consequences of not delaying childbearing past adolescence:

- Children of teen mothers are at higher risk of being of low birth weight, have lower cognitive attainment, have lower academic achievement, and exhibit greater behavioral problems.
- The sons of teen mothers are significantly more likely to be incarcerated for some time.
- The daughters of teen mothers are significantly more likely to become teen mothers themselves.
- Men who father children of teen mothers have diminished lifetime earnings.

■ Teen mothers are over twice as likely to have a report of child abuse or neglect and to have a child placed in foster care within years of birth.

In addition to the costs borne by teen mothers themselves and their children are continuing high costs to the larger society. These include expenditures responding to poor social and economic outcomes, as well as lost tax revenue from foregone earnings. Hoffman and Maynard estimate the cost to taxpayers to be $7.3 billion per year. To the extent that these high costs could be avoided, the urgency of preventing early pregnancy and parenthood remains a moral and pragmatic imperative.

Based on the most reliable existing research, this second edition retains the same organization and conceptual framework of the first edition: the fundamental dynamics of teens' sexual lives have not changed much since 2003. However, in response to recent research and lessons from relevant practice, this edition includes the following major changes:

1. A significant body of evaluation research on abstinence-only education is now available and incorporated into discussions of pregnancy prevention approaches. It is likely that political changes accompanying the new Democratic administration will shift public investment away from singular support for abstinence-only education, but decisions about which approaches to use should rest on balanced and objective analysis of available evidence of impact.
2. There is now a separate chapter on secondary prevention of teen pregnancy. Although the empirical base remains frustratingly weak as a guide to practice, the most current findings are included.
3. There is more attention paid to sexually transmitted infections throughout. Because the risks of HIV/AIDS face more young people, it is increasingly important to include sexually transmitted infection (STI) prevention as prevention goals. Thus, there is more emphasis on reducing high-risk sexual behavior as a broad perspective.
4. Findings from previous research have been updated to confirm or replace earlier conclusions throughout.
5. Policies have been updated to reflect the current status as of the time of publication.

The message remains the same: the lives of adolescents are so complex, in some ways ever more so, that our collective efforts to help them reach adulthood safely must likewise be complex and be targeted according to the sources of such complexity and diversity. Success in this endeavor is costly not only in material but perhaps even more in human resources. However, it is those human resources in the form of attention, time, and contact with young people that will make the difference in their lives and, ultimately, in the quality of all our lives.

Acknowledgments

I want to thank Susan Brower and Adair Gindar for their assistance in gathering current research findings. Katie Matheson went above and beyond reasonable expectations of a graduate assistant in each aspect of her contributions to this second edition. I am especially grateful to Candice Morgan, who provided not only dedicated assistance in research but also served as a thoughtfully critical sounding board. Finally, I want to thank Jennifer Perillo for her enthusiastic support and Brian O'Connor for his patient and ongoing help completing this work.

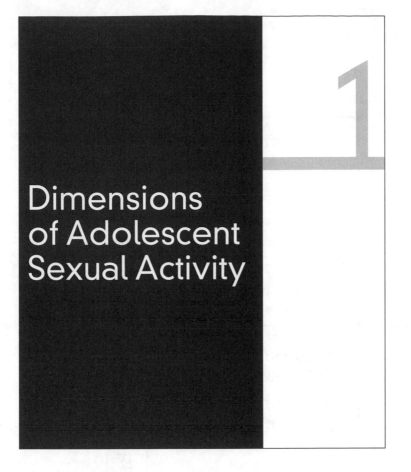

Dimensions of Adolescent Sexual Activity

Teenage pregnancy and parenthood are by no means new occurrences in the United States. However, in the past 50 years the social and economic contexts in which unmarried young people become sexually active, conceive, make decisions about pregnancy resolution, and become parents have changed dramatically. Such changes lead us today to regard these behaviors and their consequences among adolescents as sufficiently serious social problems to require intensive and formal public intervention.

During the last several decades, significant attention and resources were directed toward preventing pregnancy among teenagers with some positive effect (Brindis, 2006). Since the early 1990s (see Figure 1.1), pregnancy and childbearing among adolescents have declined by about one third. The birthrate among adolescents fell from 61.8 per 1,000 girls in 1991 to 40.4

1.1

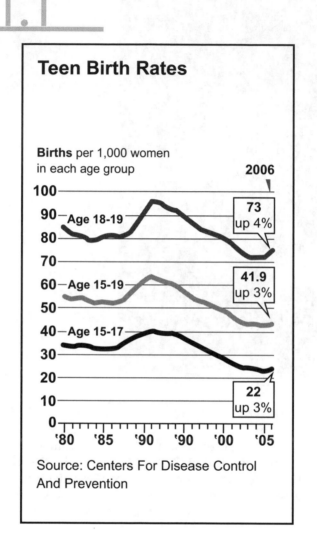

Teen Birth Rates

Births per 1,000 women
in each age group

2006

Source: Centers For Disease Control
And Prevention

in 2005, which is the lowest recorded rate in 65 years. Though the overall decrease in adolescent fertility is unambiguously good news, the positive trend halted in 2006, when the rates of childbearing among American teenagers increased for the first time since before 1991. Recent information shows that the birthrate for U.S. teenagers, age 15–19 years, rose 3% to 41.9 births per 1,000 girls between 2005 and 2006, and then rose again by 1% in 2007. The birthrate for teenagers age 15–17 years rose 3% to 22.0 per 1,000 in 2006, and 1% more to 22.2 per 1,000 in 2007. The birthrate for teenagers age 18–19 years increased 4% to 73.0 per 1,000 in 2006 and rose another 1% in 2007 to 73.9 per 1,000 girls. The youngest teenagers, age 10–14 years, were the only age group younger than 20 years whose birthrate did not increase in 2006 and 2007 (Martin et al., 2009; Hamilton, et al., 2009).

As adolescent fertility continued to decline after 1991, rates of marriage among childbearing teens also fell unabated (Ventura, 2008). The rise in childbearing outside of marriage is a crucial aspect of how the "problem" of teen pregnancy has changed over time. The individual and social costs of teen pregnancy and childbearing increasingly result from disadvantaged unmarried young women choosing to keep and raise their children, often with compromised means for supporting and nurturing them.

An examination of fertility patterns among young women over time shows that as rates fall, they also can—and do—rise. In addition, teen pregnancy and childbearing in the United States remain the highest among industrialized western countries (Figure 1.2).

In light of recent reversal of progress, continued high rates relative to other industrialized nations, and an estimated annual cost related to teen fertility of about $9.1 billion to American society, we must not be complacent about having finally solved the problems of early pregnancy and parenthood (Hoffman, 2006). This caveat is especially important because no one is certain precisely what caused the welcome changes in youths' behavior between 1991 and 2005, or what accounts for the reversal in the trend. It is extremely difficult to pinpoint exactly how much any one factor contributes to changes in such complex behaviors. Probably, the confluence of several intersecting trends in our society influenced rates of teenage pregnancy and childbearing downward and then upward again. There are, however, some identifiable correlates and plausible factors.

The immediate causes of the decline in rates of teen pregnancy and childbearing were the lower levels of sexual activity among adolescents coupled with greater use of effective contraceptives by those having sexual intercourse. These shifts were likely caused by youths having greater awareness of and concern over the dangers of contracting HIV/AIDS and other sexually transmitted infections (STIs), a generally

1.2

Rates of Teenage Pregnancy Among Industrialized Countries

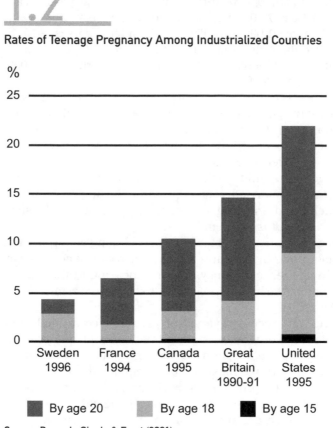

Source: Darroch, Singh, & Frost (2001).

more cautious attitude toward sexual activity among young people, a better economy, aggressive public service media campaigns, and myriad prevention programs ranging from sex education in public schools to comprehensive community-based programs that proliferated nationwide. Some observers believe that these factors and others may have created more socially conservative norms regarding sexual activity among adolescents (Sawhill & Hutchins, 2000).

It is too soon to know the meaning of the recent plateau and then rise in adolescent pregnancy and childbearing. It will be necessary to watch fertility patterns closely to determine whether increased fertility is simply an anomaly that will be reversed in the near future or is the beginning of a trend toward higher levels. It appears that rising levels of sexual activity among adolescents, coupled with small declines in contraceptive use by sexually active high school females are contributing to the upward change in fertility (Moore, 2008). What accounts for the current shifts? Just as a strong economy may indirectly contribute to decreased adolescent fertility, the present weak economy may be pushing adolescents' fertility upward. For example, the sharp spike in childbearing among high school students in Gloucester, MA that caused an international flurry of media attention based on rumors of a "pregnancy pact" in 2008 occurred in the context of a depressed local economy. One report attributes increases in teens' fertility to a loss of momentum in prevention efforts, so-called *prevention fatigue* (Moore, 2008). It may also be that the deeper cultural characteristics of American society that have contributed to relatively high levels of adolescents engaging in unprotected sex create a barrier to further significant reduction in fertility rates. That is, there may be a "floor" beneath which adolescents' fertility rates will not easily drop.

Despite the challenge of pinpointing the exact contribution of any one factor, it is clear that behind the notable decrease and then recent increase in fertility and the continuing high rate of out-of-wedlock childbearing among teenagers lay several distinct but intertwined trends. To better understand the current patterns, help sustain the positive ones, and ameliorate the more worrisome ones, it is important to examine in greater detail the fertility-related patterns of adolescents and how their context and social meanings have changed over time.

Historical Background

The definition of teenage pregnancy and childbearing as social problems per se is relatively new. The scant historical evidence suggests that young people were sexually active in earlier times, but neither sex among teenagers nor a resulting pregnancy were regarded as special problems related to their age. Rather, the history of adolescent pregnancy and childbearing as social problems in the United States is properly understood as the history of out-of-wedlock childbearing. That is, it has been primarily the meaning we attach to nonmarital sex and childbearing and their changing consequences rather than the age at which young people engage in sexual relations that has most influenced our response to teenage pregnancy.

It is not possible to determine directly historical patterns of sexual activity and conception among adolescents. Until fairly recently, most women of any age who became pregnant out of wedlock got married. Therefore, a reasonable proxy for premarital sexual activity is the incidence of premarital pregnancies, determined by measuring the time between marriage and the birth of a first child to a woman. There have been wide fluctuations in the incidence of premarital conception over the past few hundred years in the United States and Europe. The seminal research of Smith and Hindus (1975) found a range in premarital conceptions in the United States over time, from under 10% of first births in the 17th century to a high of nearly 30% in the late 18th century.

While premarital sex apparently was common in England during the 15th and 16th centuries, it declined in early Colonial America under the Puritan influence (Vinovskis, 1988). Contrary to the popular characterization of the New England Puritans as discouraging the expression of sexuality, they believed that it was an important aspect of married relations:

> . . .the Puritan attitude toward sex, though directed by a belief in absolute God-given moral values, never neglected human nature. The rules of conduct which the Puritans regarded as divinely ordained had been formulated for men, not for angels and not for beasts. God had created mankind in two sexes; He had ordained marriage as desirable for all, and sexual intercourse as essential to marriage. On the other hand, He had forbidden sexual intercourse outside of marriage. (Morgan, 1983, p. 319)

These expectations were reinforced by publicly punishing offenders and stringently enforcing paternal support of all offspring.

As sexual intimacy became more accepted as part of courting behavior during the 1700s, premarital pregnancies increased. By the end of the 18th century, social sanctions against premarital sex diminished even more, with a corresponding rise in premarital conception. In the second half of the 1700s, upward of one third of pregnancies were conceived before marriage. "This increase in premarital pregnancy paralleled a steady, visible erosion of church and civil opposition to premarital sexual activity. Across New England the number of civil prosecutions for fornication declined, as did parents' ability to persuade their children to marry partners of the parents' choosing. Without opposition from the church, civil authorities and community, sexual intimacy became a normal part of most courtships" (Harari & Vinovskis, 1993, p. 27).

One of the continuing debates in the history of nonmarital sexual behavior in the United States is why there was a subsequently dramatic decline of premarital conceptions in the mid-19th century. Vinovskis suggests that, unlike the reliance on public censure during early colonial times, in the 1800s "reformers devoted more of their efforts to instilling the values of self-control and self-discipline" (Vinovskis, 1988, p. 15). Smith and Hindus (1975) locate the heightened moral conservatism in a "new social matrix" (p. 550). This matrix was characterized by greater independence for youth at earlier ages, the economic shift from the apprentice to wage labor system, greater involvement of youth in the church, including wider participation by members of more sexually permissive classes who consequently were influenced by religious opposition to premarital sex. Smith and Hindus contend that "women also became more active and influential in church affairs and reinforced norms of nonmarital sexual abstinence" (p. 551).

"Social pressure against premarital sexual activity was not directed specifically at adolescents, despite the appearance during the 19th century of medical writings that warned of the particularly harmful effect of premarital sexual activity, including masturbation, on youthful vigor" (Harari & Vinovskis, 1993, p. 28). In general, until well into the 20th century, little attention was paid to nonmarital sexual activity among adolescents as distinct from that of any adults outside of marriage. There are several reasons for this lack of focus on teenagers. One common explanation is that in earlier times, adolescence was not defined as a discrete social phase of development. Historians of the family continue to debate to what degree Americans in the past made sharp distinctions among older children, adolescents, and adults in terms of their normative roles and expected behaviors (Demos & Boocock, 1978). Juster and Vinovskis suggest that, "it appears that in the seventeenth, eighteenth, and nineteenth century contemporaries only loosely defined the teenage years and based their observations more on economic and social status rather than chronological age" (Vinovskis, 1987, p. 206). That is, individuals' developmental maturity regarding sexuality, marriage, and parenthood were viewed less in terms of years and more in regard to their ability to fulfill adult roles.

Another reason for the absence of explicit attention to adolescents' sexual activity is that the vast majority of nonmarital conceptions were legitimated by marriage. Of course, unmarried young women did become pregnant, but as long as marriage occurred subsequently and provided for the economic support of the young mother and child, there were few negative consequences of early pregnancy. In addition, by the mid-1800s, both boys and girls usually had completed their education at the age of 15 or 16, so pregnancy did not endanger an adolescent's educational attainment as it does today.

Likewise, early marriage was not regarded as especially detrimental to women's well-being, though it was not encouraged. In Colonial America, women generally did not marry until their early 20s, the average age of marriage rising to 24 by the mid-1800s. As most women did not work for wages outside of the home, young motherhood and marriage did not derail their potential for individual economic achievement. Since divorce was relatively uncommon until recent decades, teenage pregnancy also was not associated with subsequent marital dissolution (Harari & Vinovskis, 1993). Consequently, "Although parents and community leaders discouraged premarital sexual activity and adolescent marriage and childbearing, these became disastrous only if the young couple could not support themselves and their child" (Harari & Vinovsksis, 1993, p. 29).

The cyclical pattern of premarital conceptions continued as rates rose dramatically over the second half of the 19th century, dropped again precipitously at the turn of the 20th century, and then rose for some years. The pioneering work of Alfred Kinsey during the 1940s and 1950s provides more direct information about sexual activity among young women during the first half of the 20th century. Despite the limitations of this data based on a fairly homogeneous sample of white and middle-class Americans, the changes in sexual behavior over time that he documented give an important perspective on broader changes in society. Kinsey compared patterns of premarital petting and intercourse among women born before and after 1900. He found that younger women had more sexual experience, including petting and intercourse, at earlier ages than did those women born before 1900. For example, among women who were not married by the age of 25, 14% of the "older generation" had had sexual intercourse compared to 36% of women born after 1900 (Harari & Vinovskis, 1993).

As in earlier times, nonmarital sexual relations during the early 1900s tended to occur between women and their fiancés as part of courtship leading to marriage. However, important shifts were occurring in relations within the family and among young people that resulted in less parental control of teenagers' sexual activities. On the one hand, there was more acceptance of young women having sexual experience outside of marriage and more openness about sexuality. By the 1920s, unchaperoned dating became more common. Contributing to increasing autonomy for youth, ". . .social workers and psychologists now encouraged parents to allow children more freedom from interference and free time to spend with their peers. They also instructed parents to be emotionally expressive toward their children. The new 'compassionate family' was small and placed increased importance on love and companionship between spouses and between parents and their children" (Harari & Vinovskis, 1993, p. 31). This pattern became part of the increasing separation of sex from the expectation of marriage. While in the past, some young people who were not married certainly engaged in sexual intercourse, generally it preceded marriage, by design or necessity.

On the other hand, more young women became vulnerable to the unintended consequences of the loosening of traditional gender-based double standards for sexual activity. Despite liberalization of norms regarding nonmarital sexual activity, Kinsey observed that young women did not have ready sources of information about sexuality that would help protect them from unwanted pregnancy. He "noted the absence of socialized roles for the mother, the family, the church, or the school to play in helping girls prepare for sexual relations. Instead, petting itself gave girls their 'first real understanding of heterosexual experience'" (Harari & Vinovskis, 1993, p. 32).

The Depression brought a steep decline in birthrates to adolescents. However, after World War II rates climbed again significantly and continued upward through the 1950s: "the highest rates of teenage births of the 20th century occurred in 1957, at 97.3 births per 1,000 girls aged 15–19." Birthrates fell steadily during the 1960s, taking a slight upward swing during the last couple years of the decade. It was at this time that teenage pregnancy for the first time became the subject of a focused and growing body of research and of serious consideration in the arena of public policy.

Although the actual rates of pregnancy and childbearing among adolescents have been consistently lower than in 1957, the dramatic changes in our society, since the 1950s, have profoundly altered the consequences of teenagers becoming sexually active and pregnant. As recently as a few decades ago, early sexual intercourse might simply hasten what was an expected and normative outcome for the majority of young women, marriage and motherhood. Over the last 50 years, however, as better methods of birth control have helped disconnect sex from the risk of pregnancy, sex and increasingly childbearing have also been disconnected from marriage. This severing of sex and procreation from marriage is part of significant recent behavioral and biological changes among adolescents as among older women; currently, more than one third of all children are born to unmarried mothers in the United States. Nevertheless, fertility trends among younger resulted in the intense public outcry over what some have named an "epidemic" of adolescent pregnancy. Next, we will examine more recent trends in sexual and reproductive choices in terms of their broad demographic variables.

Recent Trends in Adolescent Sexuality and Fertility

Age of Puberty

An adolescent's risk of conceiving results from both physiological and behavioral characteristics (Dunbar, Sheeder, Lezotte, Dabelea, & Stevens-Simon, 2006). To become pregnant, a young woman must be both sexually active and biologically mature enough to be fertile. The average age of sexual maturity among girls—the onset of menarche—has been declining steadily over the past 200 years (Bellis, Downing, & Ashton, 2006; Herman–Giddens, Kaplowitz, & Wasserman, 2004). Sun, Schubert, Liang, Roche, Kulin, & Lee, 2005). While there is no complete agreement among scientists about the magnitude of such change, some writers estimate the decrease in age to be as rapid as 3–4 months every decade (Zabin & Hayward, 1993; Sun, Schubert, Liang, Roche, Kulin, & Lee, et al, 2005; Herman-Giddens, Kaplowitz, & Wasserman, 2004). Today, the median age of menarche in the United States is 12.6 years. One significant implication of change in the age of menarche is that earlier physical maturation combined with later marriage, the median age for women being 25.3, and greater sexual activity result in more young women facing a longer period of risk of pregnancy outside of marriage during adolescence than teens did in the past.

There is a complex relationship between menarche, physiological capacity to conceive, and sexual activity that is not well understood. It is widely accepted that better nutrition and higher body weight contribute to the earlier onset of menarche today. Selected other factors hypothesized to account for earlier sexual development include greater consumption of hormone-laden cow's milk concomitant with a decline in breastfeeding by infants, greater environmental exposure to estrogens and endocrines, and older maternal age at childbirth (Zabin & Hayward, 1993).

There continues to be controversy over the nature of differences by race in the age of menarche (Chumlea, Schubert, Roche, Kulin, Lee, Himes and Sun, 2003; Wu, Mendola, & Buck, 2002; Anderson, Gerard, Dallal, & Must, 2003). Some researchers have found that African American girls develop secondary sexual characteristics (such as breasts and pubic hair) earlier than white girls. It appears, however, that social and economic elements are probably the major mediating factors in these small observed differences, and such interracial differences are quite minor when compared with differences between women in the United States and in less affluent nations (e.g., in Africa).

The start of puberty is marked by many aspects of physiological change that exert differential influences on the psychosexual development of both boys and girls. Zabin and Hayward (1993) summarize the processes and their social significance:

> *Pubertal development is caused by increasing levels of ste-roidal hormones. In males, all physical and morphological changes, as well as nocturnal emission and other aspects of maturation, are caused by androgens. In females, estrogens are responsible for morphological changes such as breast development and genital maturation, whereas androgens cause hair growth. . .In both sexes, androgens are respon-sible for increased sex drive experienced during the adoles-cent years. . .the role of estrogens in sexual motivation is as yet uncertain. . .The decline in mean age of menarche in the modern era means at the very least that all these changes occur at younger ages and that fertility is achieved earlier than before. And when they occur at younger ages, they create a discontinuity between biological maturity, on the one hand, and psychosocial and cognitive development, on the other. We have noted that each of these developmental processes pro-ceeds independently. One effect of earlier physical maturation is to put the young person at greater risk of conception and sexually transmitted diseases before the skills to manage a sexual life are well developed. (p. 31)*

There is not a direct relationship between when any par-ticular young woman or man reaches puberty and how likely he or she is to engage in sex or, if sexually active, to conceive. For individual young people, the interplay between their sociocultural environments and physical and psychologi-cal characteristics present various pressures, opportunities, constraints, and imperatives that influence sexual behavior and susceptibility to early pregnancy. At the same time, it is worth noting some general observations about the signifi-cance of physiological development as a risk factor for early sexual onset, especially among girls.

The actual age of physical development appears to exert a stronger influence on sexual behavior when teens are young-er. This is suggested by findings that by the age of 13, almost 40% of girls who reached menarche at the age of 11 or younger are sexually active, whereas only 10% of girls whose menarche had not occurred by the age of 14 are sexually active (Zabin & Hayward, 1993). Not until the age of 17 does this differential disappear. At the age of 11, more than half of boys who have had their first wet dream (a significant marker of advancing hormonal development) are sexually active, the differential disappearing by the age of 15. Although the association between reaching physical maturation and sexual onset does not hold throughout the teenage years, the strong relationship in earliest adolescence unfortunately brings particular risk of pregnancy, in part because younger teens do not use contraception well and they are also at higher risk of experiencing sexual coercion.

Despite the association between early physical development and sexual initiation across gender, it appears that boys and girls respond differentially to hormonal changes. The best predictor of boys' sexual behavior—both coital and noncoital—is hormonal level. For girls, noncoital sexual activity but not intercourse is related to their hormonal levels (Zabin & Hayward, 1993). Whether or not girls engage in intercourse is more dependent on their social environment, the prevailing norms, values, and attitudes about sex. Of course, boys often experience both the intense physical surge and more positive cultural messages about having sex than do girls. Nevertheless, girls' sexual onset is believed to be more socially than physically influenced, while boys seem to be responding to the intensity of dramatic hormonal change.

Sexual Initiation and Activity

It is difficult to make meaningfully precise comparisons of teens' sexual activity across time because sources of data often include different age groups, samples, and even definitions of behavior. However, it is certainly possible to chart trends and, in recent years, more narrowly defined categories of behavior by age (Whitbeck, Yoder, Hoyt, & Conger, 1999). We find that during the mid-to-late 1950s, fewer than 10% of teenage girls had had intercourse by the age of 16. Between 1971 and 1979, nationwide, "the percent of sexually active girls aged 15–19 rose significantly from 28%–46%" (Hayes, 1987, p. 40). From 1979 to 1982, there was a small decrease, followed by a steady rise over the 1980s (Zabin & Hayward, 1993). In the late 1980s, the proportion had risen to 21%; and by the 1990s, over 50% of teenage girls had had intercourse (Singh & Darroch, 1999). By 1994, the rates had risen to the modern peak of 56% among girls and to 73% among boys (The Alan Guttmacher Institute, 1999).

As the century closed, this trend reversed downward; in 1999, one half of all 9th to 12th grade students reported having had sexual intercourse, with boys only slightly more likely than girls to have become sexually active (Kaiser Family Foundation, 2000). Based on nationally representative data (rather than a sample of high school students), Hoffman and Maynard (2008) report that the percent of never-married girls who had ever had sexual intercourse before the age of 19 fell from 77% in 1988 to 70% in 1995 and remained at 70% in 2002; those girls reporting ever having intercourse by the age of 17 rose from 38% in 1988 to 47% in 1996 and fell to 43% in 2002. Boys in the same sample report even more marked changes in rates of ever having had intercourse by the age of 19: 75% in 1988 to 83% in 1995 falling significantly to 39% in 2002. Those boys reporting sexual initiation by the age of 17 remained at 53% between 1988 and 1995, then fell to 39% in 2002.

In sum, after 1995 there was a general rise in the age at first sexual experience and a decline in the proportion of teens becoming sexually active Currently, about one half of teenagers report having had sexual intercourse some time (Kirby, 2007; Kaiser Family Foundation, 2008). Rates of adolescents becoming sexually active vary by race and ethnicity: 68% of African American, 51% of nonwhite Hispanic, and 43% of white high school students report ever having had intercourse (Kirby, 2007).

Recent research shows that many adolescents believe that oral sex carries less risk than vaginal intercourse. More than half of boys and girls ages 15–19 report that they had oral sex with someone of the opposite sex (Kaiser Family Foundation, 2008). Nearly a quarter of boys and girls have had oral but not vaginal sex.

At present, the median age of first intercourse among all teenagers is 17.4 for girls and 16.9 for boys (Kaiser Family Foundation, 2008). While historically, African American youth tended to initiate sexual activity earlier than white and Hispanic youth, this gap has narrowed as non-African American teens began to have sex at younger ages. According to the Kaiser Foundation, "The percentage of 9th–12th grade students who had initiated sexual intercourse before the age of 13 has fluctuated in recent years, from 9% in 1955 (the first year data was collected) to 7.2% in 1997. This trend continues with reports of 6% girls and 8% boys initiating sex before the

the age of 14 in 2002" (Kaiser Family Foundation, 2005). The convergence among white, African American, and Hispanic youths in their likelihood of early sexual activity has been one of the most significant changes in sexual behavior in recent years (Christopher, Johnson, & Roosa, 1994; Zabin & Hayward, 1993). Nevertheless, there remain differences by race and ethnicity not only regarding whether young people become sexually active as an adolescent, but also in how early their sexual debut occurs: 16% of African American students, 8% of Latino students, and 4% of white students initiate sex before the age of 13 (Kaiser Family Foundation, 2008).

In addition to differences by race and ethnicity in early initiation of sexual activity, there are differences by socioeconomic status that appear to be independent of race or ethnicity (Santelli, Lowry, Brener, & Robin, 2000). Living in poverty is strongly associated with beginning to be sexually active as an adolescent. The significance of economic status is evident in different patterns of sexual activity by neighborhood of residence:

> In neighborhoods (defined here as block groups) with a median family income less than $20,000, 69 percent of teenage females had ever had sexual intercourse; in neighborhoods in which the median family income was between $20,000 and $50,000, 51 percent had ever had intercourse; and in neighborhoods with median family incomes of $50,000 or more, only 37 percent had ever had intercourse. . .These differences are found for both white and black teenagers. (*Ventura, Mosher, Curtin, Abma & Henshaw, 2000, p. 18*)

There is also a strong association between higher levels of sexual initiation among teenagers and higher levels of unemployment and receipt of public welfare in neighborhoods. Although the income-related gap is closing, there remains a clear relationship between low socioeconomic status (SES) and early sexual activity.

Age is also strongly related to becoming sexually active: the older the teen, the more likely he or she is to have had intercourse. The 1999 Youth Risk Behavior Survey found that between grades 9 and 12, the percentage of girls who had had sexual intercourse increased from 32.5–65.8; and among the boys, the increase was from 44.5–63.9 (CDC, 2000). A 2006 report suggests that even among teens who do become sexually active, they are waiting longer than in previous decades: 13% of girls and 15% of boys aged 15–19 in 2002 had had sex before the age of 15, compared with 19% and 21%, respectively, in 1995 (Guttmacher Institute, 2006).

Young teens and preteens face special risks when they become sexually active. Developmental characteristics typically associated with their age diminish their abilities to protect themselves against pregnancy and disease. Another critical aspect of their vulnerability has to do with the circumstances of their becoming sexually active. There is disturbing evidence that many girls younger than the age of 15 who are sexually active experienced some degree of coercion the first time they had intercourse. About 18%–24% of girls who began to have sex younger than at the age of 14 say that it was involuntary and 27% characterized their first sexual experience as unwanted (Kirby, 2007; Hoffman & Maynard, 2008). Having sex at a young age with considerably older partners increases the risk that their first sexual experiences are involuntary or unwanted (National Campaign, 2007). In addition to the potential emotional consequences of early sex in unfavorable circumstances, younger teens who experience unwanted sex are at particularly high risk for STIs and pregnancies.

The very question of whether sex is "wanted" is complex for both boys and girls throughout adolescence. Twenty percent of teens feel pressured—11% "a lot" and 26% "some"—about sex and relationships. Over one third of teens aged 13–18 report having done something sexual, or felt pressure to do something sexual that they did not feel ready to do; while almost one in ten 9th- to 12th-grade students report having ever been forced to have sexual intercourse when they did not want to—11% of girls and 5% of boys (Kaiser Family Foundation, 2008). One study found that fully 40%t of a sample of urban teenage girls reported having unwanted sex (Blythe et al., 2006). Continuing trends over the past 2 decades, involuntary sex is more common when there is a larger age gap between partners and among Hispanic and non-Hispanic African American youth (Hoffman & Maynard, 2008).

Most sexually active teenage girls, over 59%, have a first sexual partner who is 1–3 years her senior (Guttmacher Institute, 2006). The younger a girl is when she has intercourse for the first time, the greater the age difference is likely to be between her and her partner (Kaiser Family Foundation, 2000). It is not surprising, then, that upward of two thirds of fathers are estimated to be 4–6 years older than the teen mothers whom they impregnated. This age gap tends to be greater among white than among African American or Hispanic teenage mothers.

Once becoming sexually active, adolescents tend to have intercourse less frequently than do adults and many are regularly abstinent for periods of time. Among girls who are sexually active, less than half report having intercourse in the past year and a little over a third had sex in the past 3 months (Abama, Martinez, Mosher, & Dawson, 2004). In 2007, 35% of all high school students reported that they had sex with one or more people in the past 3 months (The National Campaign to Prevent Teen Pregnancy, 2008). About half of sexually experienced 14-year-old teens have had sex 0–2 times in the past 12 months. Young men (31%) are more likely than young women (24%) to report that they are currently abstinent (Kaiser Family Foundation, 2000). In general, levels of sexual activity increase with age, with older teens reporting having sex more often and having shorter periods of abstinence.

Sexual relationships among adolescents tend to be episodic and of short duration. Thus, it is common for teens to have multiple sexual partners throughout their adolescence, particularly when they initiate sexual activity at an early age. Usually, teens do not have more than one sexual partner at a time; the majority practice serial monogamy. There was a decline among 9th- to 12th-grade students who reported having four or more sexual partners, from 18% in 1995 to 15% in 2007 (Kaiser Family Foundation, 2008).

There are differences by race and gender in adolescents' patterns of sexual activity and partnering. Twenty-eight percent of non-Hispanic African American students report that they have had 4 or more sexual partners compared to 17% of Hispanic and 12% of white students (The National Campaign to Prevent Teenage Pregnancy, 2008). These differences are accounted for partly by how early teens in each groups initiate sexual activity. The greater the number of partners with whom a teen is sexually intimate, whether serially or simultaneously, the higher the teen's risk of contracting—and passing on—STIs. Consequently, reducing the number of partners among sexually active teens is an important objective for their own health and those of potential members of their and their partners' sexual networks.

Contraceptive Use

Although adolescents' rates of pregnancy rose overall between 1970 and 1990, their more effective use of birth control helped minimize the increase and continues to mitigate the impact of high levels of sexual activity on pregnancy rates. That is, without a concomitant increase in contraception, the rate of teenage pregnancies would have been and remained higher. One study estimates that over one million pregnancies were avoided by teenagers using birth control (Kahn, Brindis, & Glei, 1999; Glei, 1999). Today, most sexually active teens report that they use birth control at least sometimes. Nevertheless, despite the rise in teens' use of birth control, studies documenting this increase do not always reveal the complexity of measuring actual pattern of use. The challenge in capturing accurate information likely results in underestimating how inconsistent teenagers are in their real use of birth control over time.

Between the early 80s and mid-90s, the use of contraception by sexually active teens declined. The percent of teens who used contraception both the first time and most recent time they had sex fell, then subsequently rose. Current research finds that about 74% of girls used birth control the first time they had sex and 83% during the most recent sexual encounter. Boys report even higher levels of contraception, 82% the first time they had sex and 90% the last time they had intercourse (Kirby, 2007).

Overall rates of contraceptive use vary widely among sexually active teens according to their race and ethnicity. Hispanic teens are less likely than African American or white teens to use birth control at first intercourse or any time thereafter. Among Hispanic youth, 73% of boys and 66% of girls report using a method of contraception at first intercourse, in contrast to 85% of white boys and 78% of white girls and 86% of African American boys and 71% of African American girls (National Campaign to Prevent Pregnancy, 2006).

In recent years, sexually active teens have changed not only their propensity to use contraception but the methods they choose. The most commonly used method of birth control among teens is the condom. Condom use by 15- to 19-year-old teens at first intercourse rose from 69% to 71% between 1995 and 2002 (Guttmacher Institute, 2008). In 2007, 62% of sexually active high school students used a condom the last time they had sex (Kaiser Family Foundation, 2008). This includes 69% of African American, 63% of white, and 58% of Hispanic students. Although condoms have about a 97% success rate when used properly, the American Academy of Family Physicians estimates that "typical" use of condoms by teenagers results in a 14% failure rate (As–Sanie, Gantt, & Rosenthal, 2004). Nevertheless, even imperfect use of condoms contributes to teens protecting themselves and their partners from pregnancy and STIs.

After condoms, the next most frequently used form of contraception is the pill. About 16% of sexually active high school students report that they or their partner were using an oral contraception at last intercourse (Kaiser Family Foundation, 2008). White students are twice as likely as African Americans or Hispanics to use an oral contraceptive. Oral contraception is extremely effective in preventing pregnancy, with a less than 1% failure rate when used as prescribed (As–Sanie et al., 2004). However, it is important to note that even when a young woman says that she used birth control at last intercourse or that she currently "uses" the birth control pill, it is not uncommon to miss taking her contraceptive pill 1 day and then double up the next day, leaving her unprotected from pregnancy. Some research finds that among 15- to 19-year-old girls relying upon oral contraceptives, only 70% take the pill everyday (National Campaign to Prevent Teen Pregnancy, 2007). Teenagers who recently began to use the pill and those who have already had one unplanned pregnancy are especially inconsistent in their use.

A rising minority of sexually active girls use injectable and other nonoral forms of hormonal birth control, such as Depo-Provera or the contraceptive patch (Dinerman, Wilson, Duggan, &,1995). Like oral contraceptives, these other hormonal methods are over 99% effective when used properly. They have the important advantage over all other types of birth control of requiring relatively infrequent doses. These methods range from the Ortho Evra patch that requires weekly application for 3 out of 4 weeks per month, to the single-rod implant that lasts for 3 years, to intrauterine devices (IUDs) that can remain in place for up to 10 years. Almost 10% of teens used

1.3

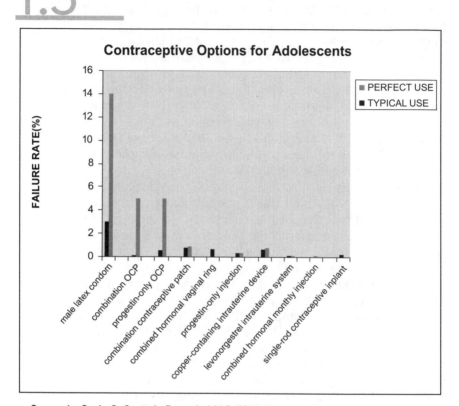

Source: As-Sanie, S., Gantt, A., Rosenthal, M.S. (2004). Pregnancy Prevention in Adolescents. *American Family Physician*,70,15 -1524.

a hormonal contraceptive at last intercourse, but over 20% of teens report that they have ever used one. Introduced in the 1990s, their use has doubled in the past decade and likely will continue to gain popularity in use (see Figure 1.3).

The rising incidence of STIs among adolescents leads most health-related professionals to recommend strongly that teens use dual methods of contraception. Best practice suggests that the best way to guard sexual health is to use hormonal birth control to prevent pregnancy and a condom to prevent an STI. Increasingly, teenage girls appear to be taking greater responsibility for prevention. The percentage of teenage girls using both a condom and hormonal contraception nearly doubled to between 1995 and 2002 to about 20% (Kaiser Family Foundation, 2008).

The rates of ever having used contraception are fairly similar among African American, white, and Hispanic teens; 97.1%, 98.4%, and 94.3% respectively. However, there are important differences by teens' race and ethnicity in the kinds of contraception they use. White students are much more likely than African American and Hispanic students to report using birth control pills before they last had sex or at all and also to use withdrawal (National Campaign to Prevent Teenage Pregnancy, 2008; Hoffman & Maynard, 2008). Condom use is high among both African American teens (94.6%) and white teens (95.9%), much less so among Hispanics (82.8%) (Hoffman & Maynard, 2008). This places sexually active Hispanic teens at disproportionately high risk for STIs. Significantly more black and Hispanic teens use injectable contraception than whites. White teens are most likely to use emergency contraception, followed by Hispanic and then African American teens. Overall, about 8% of sexually active adolescents use emergency contraception some time.

Economic status is also associated with different patterns of contraception: among girls who are sexually active, 78% of very poor teenage women, 71% of low income, and 83% of higher income report using birth control regularly (National Campaign to Prevent Teen Pregnancy, 1999). Low-income teenagers are twice as likely as more affluent teenagers to experience a pregnancy that is unplanned even while reportedly using the birth control pill or condom. One study that included estimates of "contraceptive failure rates" of teens reported that, "In general, failure rates were higher for teenagers whose family income was less than 200% of the federally defined poverty level and for those who had never been married" (Kahn et al., 1999).

Probably the most important factor in whether sexually active teenagers use birth control is their age. While younger teens are more likely than older and more sexually experienced teens to use a condom, with its dual protection against pregnancy and STI, they are also less adept and reliable in using birth control each time they have sex. The younger an adolescent is, the less likely he or she is to use contraception or to seek help in avoiding pregnancy. While teenagers generally are less effective at contraception than older women, younger teens are even less so.

Another important influence on contraceptive behavior is the nature of the relationship in which sex occurs. Teens are more likely to use a condom with a casual partner than with a steady romantic partner. However, teens in a steady relationship in general are more inclined to use effective contraception, such as hormonal methods. Recent research highlights the growing consensus that when adolescents are comfortable in a relationship and able to communicate openly about risks of STI and pregnancy with their partner, they are able to negotiate good choices about birth control (Manlove, Ryan, & Franzetta, 2007).

Teenagers who go to a physician or clinic for contraception wait for an average of 11 months after first having sex to do so. However, young teens tend to wait even longer to seek assistance. This long delay is particularly problematic because of the high risk of pregnancy in the early months after onset of sexual activity, a risk that is heightened when teens initiate sex at a younger age. When exposure to pregnancy risk starts early, the overall risk of conceiving is higher. Zabin and Hayward (1993) observe that young teens who are sexually active often appear at clinics for birth control only after they are already pregnant.

Patterns of contraception vary some among teenagers who have already had a child. African American teen mothers are significantly more likely today and more likely than other teens to use very effective contraception such as Depo-Provera or Norplant. Their use of the pill has dropped steadily and dramatically. Greater availability and use of these very effective forms of birth control certainly contributed to the decline in subsequent pregnancies among African American teen mothers over the last decade.

Rates of Adolescent Pregnancy

Between 1991 and 2005, there was a remarkable decline in the rates of pregnancies among all teenagers and among sexually active teenagers. Yet, the most recent evidence indicates that, after a few years of plateau, the trend may be reversing. In 2002, about 75 of every 1,000 girls age 15–19 became pregnant. Despite the overall downward trend in rates of conception, cumulatively, over 30% of adolescent girls still become pregnant at least once before the age of 20 (Kirby, 2007).

The decline in pregnancy rates occurred among adolescents of all ages. Among teens aged 15–17 the rate of pregnancy fell 16% from 80.3 per 1,000 in 1990 to 67.8 in 1996, and then even more dramatically to 42.3 in 2002 (Hoffman & Maynard, 2008). The rate for older teens also dropped, down 12% from 167.2 per 1,000 to 146.4 in 1996, continuing downward to 125.6 in 2002 and then to 119 in 2004 (Ventura, 2000; Hoffman & Maynard, 2008; Kaiser Family Foundation, 2008). Older teens, however, continue to have the highest incidence of pregnancy among all adolescents: about 70% of pregnancies to adolescents occur among 18–19-year olds (Kaiser Family Foundation, 2008).

Rates of teen pregnancy for all races fell, but the overall decline does not reveal the uneven changes by race and ethnicity. The drop was most dramatic among African American teens, about 40% between 1991 and 2000 (Ventura et al., 2000; Hoffman & Maynard, 2008). Pregnancy among Hispanic teens also declined but less so. In 2002, the rate of pregnancy was 48 among white girls age 15–19, 134 among African American girls, and 132 among Hispanic girls per 1,000. The differences by race and ethnicity overall are consistent among older teens ages 18–19: in 2004, pregnancy rates were 79.3 per 1,000 for whites, 202.9 for African Americans, and 210.0 for Hispanics (Ventura et al., 2008).

Another way of viewing the differences by race and ethnicity is in terms of how many teens who had intercourse in the past year became pregnant: one out of three sexually active African Americans and Hispanic teens conceived in a year compared with one out of six white teens. Among sexually active teens, then, rates of conception were 142 for whites, 305 for African Americans, and 291 per 1,000 for Hispanic youth (Ventura et al., 2000). The lower rates of pregnancy among white teens results from their being less sexually active at young ages and more likely to take measures to prevent pregnancy when they do have intercourse (Ventura et al, 2000).

It is clear that recent changes in both sexual and contraceptive behavior have had a positive impact on pregnancy rates among adolescents. The most immediately visible changes include white teens' greater use of condoms and their postponement of sexual initiation coupled with African Americans teens' use of injectable and implant birth control.

Sexually Transmitted Infections

Sexually active teenagers face significant risk of contracting STIs. Young people ages 15–24 constitute fully half of all new cases of STI, and every year there are about 4 million new cases of STI among teenagers. The CDC (2008) estimates that about one in four girls ages 14–19, about 3.2 million, is infected with at least one STI. Prevalence varies significantly by race: 48% among African American girls versus 20% among both white and Hispanic girls. In the face of this major threat to teens' immediate and long-term health, any consideration of the most effective ways to reduce teen pregnancy and child-bearing should also include reduction of STI as a corollary objective. Among the many types of STIs, the most common among adolescents are human papillomavirus (HPV), chlamydia, gonorrhea, trichomoniasis, syphilis, and HIV. These STIs vary in modes of transmission, symptoms, and health consequences. The risk of contracting an STI increases with the number of risk factors including socioeconomic status, abuse, exposure to violence, substance use, and depression (Buffardi et. al., 2008).

Human Papillomavirus (HPV). Human papillomavirus (HPV) is the most common sexually transmitted virus worldwide, including in the United States. HPV poses serious long-term risks for young women because it is associated with later development of cervical cancer. The prevalence among adolescents is about 25%. HPV can be transmitted either sexually or nonsexually, including by nonpenetrating sexual contact. Risk for contracting HPV is particularly high if girls first have sexual intercourse at a young age, and have multiple sexual partners. Younger girls are at such high risk because cervical tissue changes during puberty support the replication of HPV, thus raising the risk for active infection. High rates of infection and the health risks of HPV lead the American Cancer Society to recommend that all girls age 11–12 be vaccinated against HPV and girls and women age 13–26 receive "catch up" vaccination. This remains an extremely controversial recommendation in many communities, but does highlight the seriousness of the threat to young women's health.

Chlamydia. Chlamydia is the most frequently reported bacterial sexually transmitted disease in the United States. Among

15–19-year-old teens, rates of chlamydia infection are about 1,600 per 1000,000. Here is higher incidence among girls (2,862 per 100,000) than among boys (CDC, 2006). African American women have the highest rates of infection, followed by American Indian/Alaska Natives, Hispanic, white, and Asian/Pacific Islanders (CDC, 2006). Untreated, chlamydia can cause damage to a woman's reproductive organs and result in infertility. However, because symptoms may be mild or absent, young women often are not aware of being infected and so do not seek testing and treatment. Chlamydia is quite effectively treated with injected antibiotics, though reinfection is common.

Gonorrhea. Gonorrhea is another curable bacterial STI that occurs commonly among adolescents and young adults, second in prevalence after, and often concurrently with chlamydia. After several years of decreasing incidence, rates of gonorrhea among both boys and girls ages 15–19 increased among all races and ethnic groups except Asians in 2006. Gonorrhea, like chlamydia, is more prevalent among girls than among boys. It is spread by vaginal, oral, or anal sexual contact. Gonorrhea can spread to other parts of the body, (e.g., to the eyes) after touching infected genitals, as well as to infants from an infected mother. Boys typically experience some symptoms when they become infected, but girls less so. Though gonorrhea is very effectively treated with antibiotics, untreated infection among girls can cause pelvic inflammatory disease (PID) sterility, and ectopic pregnancy.

Trichomoniasis. Trichomoniasis is another common and readily treatable STI. Caused by the parasite, *Trichomonas vaginali*, it is the most commonly diagnosed STI among adolescents after HPV. Trichomoniasis is transmitted sexually through penis-to-vagina (or vulva-to-vulva) contact. The most common site of infection for boys is the urethra and for girls the vagina. Girls can contract the disease from an infected partner of either gender, but boys typically contract it only form infected girls.

Syphilis. Syphilis, caused by the bacterium *Treponema pallidum*, shares many of the signs and symptoms of other diseases, but over time has a distinct trajectory that, if untreated, carries distinct and serious health risks. Syphilis is contracted by both boys and girls through direct contact with a syphilis sore, typically during vaginal, anal, or oral sex. These sores occur mainly on the external genitals, vagina, anus, or in the rectum but also can occur on the lips and in the mouth. Syphilis has declined markedly among African American youth but not among white and Hispanic teens. Syphilis develops from the primary phase, marked by a sore or chancre to secondary syphilis, characterized by skin rash and mucous membrane lesions. The final and latent stage of syphilis begins after primary and secondary symptoms disappear. Ultimately, the untreated disease can result in damage to internal organs, including the brain, nerves, eyes, heart, blood vessels, liver, bones, and joints, which can cause death. As with the other sexually transmitted diseases discussed thus far, syphilis can be effectively treated when diagnosed early.

While the STIs most frequently diagnosed among adolescents are curable, there are some exceptions. For example, herpes simplex virus type 2 can be treated to reduce outbreaks of the symptoms, but not actually cured.

Most adolescents who contract a sexually transmitted illness can be successfully treated, thus providing a cure for the immediate disease and the opportunity, through behavioral changes, for prevention of further illness. HIV and AIDS present a far different set of health issues for young people. Although the prevalence of HIV/AIDS among teenagers is fairly low, the number of cases rose between 2001 and 2005 (Kirby, 2007). In 2005, among 13- to 19-year-old teens, there were 6,324 reported cases of AIDS. However, because of the potentially lengthy time between being infected with HIV and onset of AIDS, the best way to gauge current trends is through rates of HIV. Among younger teens, 77% of new HIV cases are among girls, in contrast to older teens, among whom boys are slightly more likely to be newly-infected. Girls are more likely to be infected through heterosexual contact, often with injection drug users, whereas for boys, it is more often male-to-male sexual transmission (Kirby, 2007). In 2003, about three-quarters of new infections were reported among African American youth.

There is a close connection between HIV/AIDS and other STIs that heightens the urgency of diagnosing, treating, and ultimately preventing STIs among young people: "Individuals who are infected with STDs are at least two to five times more likely than uninfected individuals to acquire HIV infection if they are exposed to the virus through sexual contact. In addition, if an HIV-infected individual is also infected with another STD, that person is more likely to transmit HIV through sexual contact than other HIV-infected persons" (Wasserheit, 1992). There appear to be two main ways through which susceptibility to getting and passing on HIV increases by having an STI. The first is through genital ulcers that break in the genital lining or skin and create a point of entry for HIV. Second, the inflammation resulting from genital ulcers or nonulcerative STDs, such as chlamydia, gonorrhea, and trichomoniasis, creates a greater concentration of cells in genital secretions that can serve as targets for HIV when they are exposed to semen or other sources of HIV (CDC, 2008). Thus, increasingly the importance of helping adolescents prevent pregnancy must be understood equally as helping them safeguard their health from potentially deadly threats.

Births to Adolescents

After several years of good news, births to teens not only stopped dropping, but they also began rising. In 2005, about 40 of every 1,000 girls between the age of 15 and 19 gave birth (Kirby, 2007). Between 2005 and 2006, birthrates among teens increased from 40.5–41.9 per 1,000 and then rose the next year to 42.5 per 1,000 teens (Hamilton, Martin, & Ventura, 2007; 2009). The rates and their pattern of change differ by race and ethnicity The birthrates per 1,000 teenagers include: 81.7 among Hispanics, 63.7 among African Americans, 59 among American Indian or Alaska Natives, and 26.6 among whites (Martin, et al., 2009). This disappointing change follows 13 years of decline in rates of adolescent childbearing.

After rates rose between 1986 and 1991, there began a steady drop throughout the 1990s and early part of this decade in the proportion of American teenagers who gave birth. In 1998, the birthrate for all teens was 51.1, 2% lower than in 1997 and 18% lower than in 1991 (Ventura et al., 2000). This reflects the lower level of sexual initiation and activity among young people and better use of birth control.

Comparing birthrates by race and ethnicity (see Figure 1.4), the largest decrease was among African American teens. Between 1991 and 1998, the birthrate for black teens aged

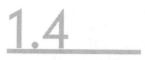

1.4

Births to Adolescents

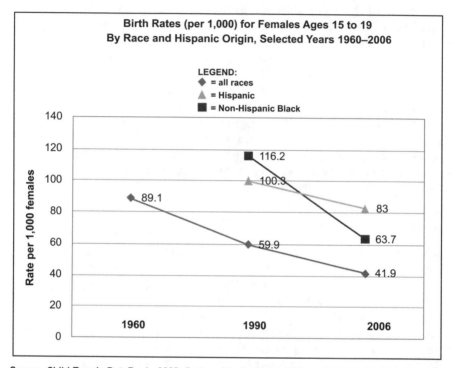

**Birth Rates (per 1,000) for Females Ages 15 to 19
By Race and Hispanic Origin, Selected Years 1960–2006**

LEGEND:
◆ = all races
▲ = Hispanic
■ = Non-Hispanic Black

Source: Child Trends DataBank, 2008, Guttmacher Institute, 2006, and Martin JA, Hamilton BE, Sutton PD, Ventura SJ, et al. Births: Final data for 2006. National vital statistics reports; vol 57 no 7. Hyattsville, MD: National Center for Health Statistics. 2009.

15–17 fell 26% from 115.5 to 85.4 (Ventura et al., 2000). This rate is the lowest for African American youths since 1960. The birthrate among Hispanic teens fell 13% between 1994 and 1998 (107.7) (National Campaign to Prevent Teen Pregnancy, 1999) Since 1994, Hispanics have had the highest birthrate among all racial and ethnic groups. However, it is important to make finer cultural distinctions within major ethnic groups. For example, the birthrate for Cuban teens increased 38.3% between 1991 and 1998, but among other major subgroups of Hispanic teens, the birthrates declined (National Campaign to Prevent Teen Pregnancy, 1999). Among Mexican Americans, the birthrate fell 4.2%; among Puerto Ricans, it fell 27.1%; and the birthrate among teens of "other/unknown" descent fell 18.2% (National Campaign to Prevent Teen Pregnancy, 1999). It is noteworthy that in the context of the last few years' rise in births to teens, only the rate to Hispanic adolescents declined, by 2%, in 2007 (Hamilton, Martin, & Ventura, 2009). Among other ethinic groups, the greatest increase over the past year was reported for American Indian or Alaska native teenagers, up 7% during 2006–2007 (Hamilton, Martin, & Ventura, 2009).

Rates of second births to teenage mothers also declined significantly between 1991 and 1997. Most dramatic was the decline of 28% in second births to African American teenage mothers from 221 to 181 per 1,000 adolescents (Ventura et al., 2000). Second births to teenage mothers are much greater than the likelihood of a first birth to teens who have not had a baby. In 2001, there were 35 births per 1,000 girls who had not previously had a baby compared with 175 births per 1,000 girls who had previously had one baby (Child Trends, 2003)

Birthrates to girls aged 15–19 also vary considerably across states, ranging from a low of 17.7 in New Hampshire to 63.4 in District of Columbia (CDC, 2008). These differences are in part related to patterns of racial and ethnic composition of each state. Generally, those states with higher proportion of African American and Hispanic teens have higher rates of teen pregnancy and childbearing. However, when comparing teen birthrates by race and ethnicity, it is important to consider the impact of poverty on patterns of early conception and childbearing.

Although birthrates declined consistently across population groups, as well as across almost all states, the overall teen birthrate is still higher than it was in the mid-1980s. In addition, in contrast to the rate of births, the actual number of births to teens in the oldest age group actually increased 3%. This is because there was a 5% increase in the number of teenage girls aged 18–19 in the general population. A broad demographic perspective is crucial in assessing the overall risk and magnitude of early childbearing in our society: even in the face of a lower proportion of youth having children, the total number of births can increase, as is occurring among Hispanic adolescents. Thus, even maintaining stable rates of pregnancy and childbearing may result in a greater number of adolescents having children in coming years, perhaps as much as a 26% increase.

Abortion

Not all teenagers' pregnancies result in a live birth. About 14% of pregnancies to adolescents end in miscarriage and about 35% are aborted (Neinstein et al., 2009). Abortions to teenagers account for about one quarter of all abortions performed nationwide, with variations by state.

During the years immediately following the legalization of abortion in 1973, abortion rates among women of all ages, including teenagers rose and then remained steady until the early 1980s. From 1988 to 1996, the abortion rate for teenagers fell 33% from 43.5 to 29.2 per 1,000 adolescents (Ventura et al., 2000). From its high, the teen abortion rate decreased by more than half by 2000 (Ventura et al., 2003). In 2004, the abortion rate for teens age 15–19 was 19.8 per 1,000 girls (Kaiser Family Foundation, 2008).

This trend is consistent with changes in attitudes of young men toward abortion. Between 1988 and 1995, approval of abortion by young men decreased significantly (Boggess & Bradner, 2000). The change was greatest among non-Hispanic whites, and coincided with an increase in the self-reported importance of religion, especially among fundamentalist Christian youth, and more conservative attitudes toward premarital sexual intercourse. Young men's perspectives on abortion are important to consider because the fathers of teens' babies often strongly influence the outcome of a young woman's pregnancy. The majority of minors who have abortions—about 61%—do so with at least one parent's knowledge and that the majority of those parents support their daughter's decision (Kaiser Family Foundation, 2000).

The abortion rate among all minority youth is considerably higher than among white teenagers. This is mainly the result of their having higher rates of sexual activity and lower use of contraception, thus being more likely to experience an unintended pregnancy. In addition, however, African American teens who are pregnant are more likely than other teens to seek an abortion: in 2004, more than 37% of pregnancies among African American teens ended in abortion, compared to 12% for whites and 19% for Hispanics (CDC, 2008).

Adoption

Although most pregnant adolescents say that they did not intend to become pregnant, most teenagers who carry their pregnancy to term choose to keep their children (Barth, 1987; Remez, 1992; Resnick, 1984; Dworkin, Harding, & Schreiber, 1993). It is difficult to obtain reliable information about formal adoption rates among teenagers. Some current estimates are that only about 9% of white and 5% of African American adolescent mothers relinquish their children, while other research indicates that less than 4% of all pregnant teens place their children for adoption (Donnelly &Voyandoff, 1991). This trend toward fewer teenagers choosing adoption to resolve an unplanned pregnancy is consistent with the decline among adult women relinquishing infants for adoption.

Young women who release children for adoption tend to be different from other pregnant teens, especially teens who choose to parent (Donnelly & Voyandoff, 1991). Young teens relinquish more often than those older than 18. Those who relinquish are more likely to be white, come from more affluent families, have higher levels of education and perceive more educational and other options besides motherhood, and have positive attitudes toward adoption. There is some evidence that young women who choose adoption are also more apt to have been sexually abused.

Births to Unmarried Adolescents

When the rate of teens bearing children was twice as high in 1957 as it is today, almost all births were legitimated by marriage—shotgun or otherwise. Today, a small minority of pregnant teens marry. Although the birthrates to teens overall and to unmarried teens have been dropping steadily in recent years, the proportion of teens who give birth and are unmarried continues to rise. This trend is part of a widespread shift in social norms regarding out-of-wedlock childbearing: today, reaching an historic high, about 40% of all births in the United States are to unmarried women, including approximately 22% among white, 43% among Hispanic, and 68% among African American women (Hamilton, Martin, & Ventura, 2009). Another way of indicating the tectonic shifts in norms of single motherhood is that in 1970 teens comprised half of all births to unmarried women. In 7 only about 23% of all births to single mothers were to adolescents (Hamilton, Martin, & Ventura, 2009).

1.5

Teen births by marital status

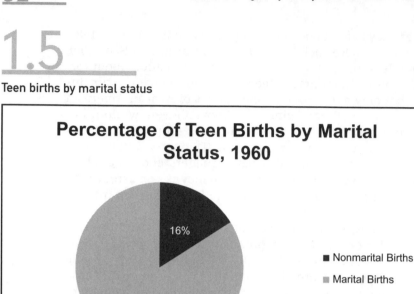

Percentage of Teen Births by Marital Status, 1960

16%

84%

- Nonmarital Births
- Marital Births

Source: U.S. Department of Health and Human Services (1995) and Ventura et. al. (1998).

Mirroring the much greater acceptance of childbearing outside of marriage and single motherhood throughout American society, the likelihood that a teenager who gives birth is married has decreased dramatically over the last 3 decades (see Figure 1.5). Nationwide, in 2004 (see Figure 1.6), over 80% of births to teens were outside of marriage (Hoffman & Maynard, 2008).

African American teenagers are least likely to marry to legitimize a birth—less than 4%. Childbearing Hispanic teenagers are still more likely than either African American or white teens to be married, about 23%, but their rates of out-of-wedlock parenthood are rising (Hoffman & Maynard, 2008). Of all major racial and ethnic groups, Asian American teenagers are least likely to bear a child outside of marriage. A notable exception to the low-birth rates among Asian American teenagers, Hmong youth have relatively high rates of fertility but also are more likely than other teens to marry (Farber, 1999).

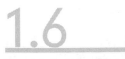

Teen births by marital status

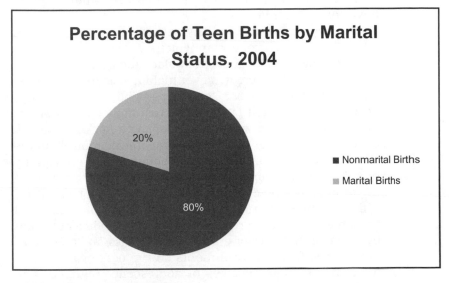

Source. Hoffman and Maynard (2008).

Summary

The second half of the last and first decade of this century have seen a profound transformation in patterns of family formation that are reflected in the contemporary sexual and reproductive behaviors of America's young people. The peak in the rates of pregnancy among adolescents occurred in the late 1950s. However, during the subsequent decades, changing social mores and a highly sexualized and individualistic youth culture resulted in many diverse groups of young men and women being vulnerable to early pregnancy and child-bearing outside of marriage. What in earlier times more often led to the formation of marital families increasingly results in single-parent, usually single-mother, families with all of the associated economic, social and psychological vulnerability experienced by both parents and children.

It is a cause of optimism that the rapidly accelerating trend toward adolescents having earlier sexual initiation and the high rates of pregnancies and births that we saw through the 1980s slowed, even declined somewhat, in certain subgroups of youths. In addition, more young men and women have greater access to and better ability to use various effective methods of birth control when they do have sexual intercourse.

At the same time, fertility rates have risen again. In addition, the social context in which ever younger boys and girls become sexually active and place themselves at risk of pregnancy and STIs creates ever higher costs for unplanned and youthful parenthood. Decreasing public interest in supporting single-parent families creates higher expectations for young women to work outside of the home. As research continues to discover more worrisome information about the short- and long-term negative consequences of growing up in a mother-only home, our sense of urgency in preventing the formation of new adolescent families should be growing. This is particularly true for those populations of youths that are already at greatest risk for the worst individual outcomes by virtue of their race or ethnicity, their class, and their community and family environments. In the next two chapters, we examine major theories of adolescent pregnancy and parenthood, and why the risks of early sexually activity, pregnancy, and parenthood vary so among youths.

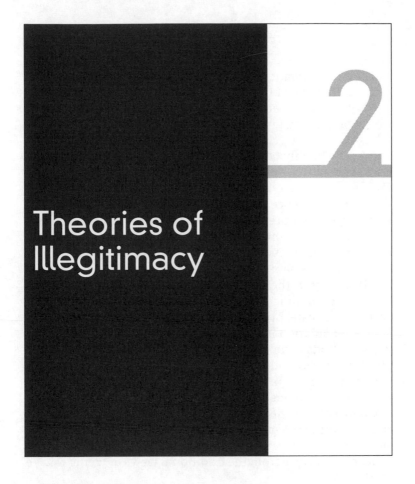

Theories of Illegitimacy

Several of the changing patterns of adolescents' sexual behavior and fertility described in chapter 1 may be summarized in the following generalizations. In comparison to past generations, more young people of diverse demographic characteristics:

- Are having sexual relations at younger ages;
- Are at increased risk for a range of serious sexually transmitted infections (STI) with potentially long-term health consequences;
- Have more types of birth control available for preventing pregnancy;
- Have more alternative pregnancy resolutions available to them;

■ Are dramatically less likely to marry to legitimize a
  nonmarital birth;
■ Choose to become a single parent rather than abort a
  pregnancy, give up the child for adoption or marry.

As the likelihood of a teenager having sex and of a pregnant teenager who bears a live infant becoming a single
mother each have grown over the years, social work and
other social science researchers have changed their understanding of teen pregnancy and parenthood. In this chapter,
we will examine the development of major theories about
why some unmarried adolescents are more likely than others
to become pregnant and bear children.

It is only in the last 50 years or so that pregnancy and
parenthood among adolescents have been defined as discrete formal categories for study and even more recently as a
special population in need of services by professional social
workers. Today the dominant conceptualization of teenage
pregnancy and childbearing views the outcome of adolescent parenthood in terms of the many complex decisions
an individual teenager makes from the time she becomes
sexually active to deciding to keep her child. Focusing on the
relative influence of specific factors on each of these decisions within a developmental perspective represents a significant departure from the traditional views of young unwed
motherhood.

Until fairly recently, it was marital status of mothers,
regardless of age, that created concern among the public and
professionals. Consistent with this attitude, most research
relevant to teen childbearing before the 1970s examined the
causes of illegitimacy per se in general as a form of social
deviance. Subsequent research has followed the perspective
advocated by Catherine Chilman in her then comprehensive
review of the research on teenage sexuality, pregnancy, and
childbearing in 1981:

> The causes of out-of-marriage childbearing are deceptively
> simple. Obviously, illegitimacy is a result of premarital
> coitus, premarital conception, lack of pregnancy interrup-
> tion, and the birth of a child before marriage. . .Complicat-
> ed questions arise in reaction to this simple formula. Why
> do some teenagers have pre-marital intercourse while
> others do not? Why do sexually active adolescents fail to

use effective contraceptives consistently? Why do so many pregnant teenagers not use abortion? Why do large numbers fail to marry if they are pregnant? In general, it is more appropriate to look for causes of illegitimacy by examining the causes of the above behaviors, rather than to look at illegitimacy as a separate entity. (Chilman, 1979, p. 199)

In keeping with this perspective, the direction of research has been away from seeking conceptually unitary and universal explanations of teen pregnancy and toward more empirically based studies intended to establish causal relationships among numerous variables and fertility outcomes. The result of this burgeoning research is a significant amount of information about which young men and women, of particular demographic and psychological characteristics, under what physical, familial, social and economic conditions are more or less likely to have sexual intercourse, how often and with how many partners, use contraception, contract an STI, become pregnant (or impregnate a girl), carry or abort a pregnancy, and remain unmarried or marry. Though the literature on adolescent sexuality is not uniformly theoretically coherent, existing information is highly useful for assessing differential levels of risk for early pregnancy and parenthood as well as STI.

The current literature that informs social work practice encompasses many more aspects of the individual adolescent and his or her environment. It also incorporates findings from a wide range of disciplines such as public health, sociology, psychology, economics, and medicine. This broad knowledge base is highly consistent with a genuinely ecological perspective on teen sexuality, pregnancy, and childbearing. Before examining contemporary literature, however, it is important to review the foundation of earlier and influential approaches to the study of illegitimacy (Blaikie, 1995).

Early Social Work Treatment of Illegitimacy

Until the ascendancy of psychoanalytic theory in social work practice during the 1940s, little research examined in detail the causes of unmarried motherhood. Social workers' primary roles with unmarried mothers were advising them about whether or not to keep their infants and assisting the women in finding respectable employment and living situations, as described in *The Family* in 1902:

> We endeavor to find out what ought to be done in the particular case. It may be to take the child from the mother and place it in a family home; it may be to secure a situation where she can nurse her baby and keep it with her; it may be to secure a boarding place where the mother can pay board; it may be to care for the mother and the child in a suitable institution; it may be to induce the grandparents to adopt the child as their own; or it may be to bring about a marriage between the parents. (Smith, 1934, p.).

Typically, unmarried women who chose to keep their infants were placed as domestic workers, with their children, if suitable. Gordon Hamilton (1923) summed up the usual methods of early social workers for various ills, including unmarried motherhood:

> Treatment, for the most part, employed a few standard remedies: the pill for poverty was work; the pill for desertion was the law or the workhouse; the pill for a kind of chronic dependency was removing people, with all due precaution, to their native locality; the pill for the unmarried mother was a place at service; the pill for broken homes and behavior problem children was, regrettable, often, the institution; the pill for many medical problems in early hospital social service was convalescent care. (p. 114)

Consistent with the primary professional focus on the disposition of a child born to an unmarried mother, the little research in the area was designed to help social workers make better-informed choices on behalf of their clients. For example, the Smith College Studies in Social Work in 1940 reported findings from a study in New York, *A Method of Predicting the Probable Disposition of Their Children by Unmarried Mothers*, based on case records from the Hebrew Home for Infants (Rome, 1940). This data was intended to be used by caseworkers in their assessments of the motivations of young unmarried mothers to place the infants permanently, temporarily, or keep them.

Social workers' concerns about unmarried mothers' rehabilitation also was consistent with the prevailing view that illegitimacy often resulted from individual moral failure.

This assumption is expressed clearly in the words of a case-worker from the Boston Children's Aid Society in 1890:

> *It is not only best that these mothers be helped to bear and not get rid of their burdens, but also equally desirable that the mothers be kept from associating with one another, and be placed under the influence of home life. . . There is, moreover, I think, nothing worse for people who have been guilty of misconduct than to find that plenty of other people have done the same thing. We can only preserve the sensitiveness of the fallen and stimulate moral sensibility and rouse them to do better by securing the maximum contact with people living under such natural and virtuous conditions such as we wish to establish in their lives. (Smith, 1934, p. 311)*

At the same time, social workers also recognized individual variability among the factors that resulted in illegitimate births. In 1910, Alice Cheyney of the Philadelphia Children's Bureau reported:

> *From the details analyzed out of individual cases I have tried to construct a composite picture. That is, I have tried to tell the general story as the record tells each individual story—with a view to the best possible reconstruction and a weather eye open for causes, in the hope that some practical remedy may be visible to prevent the repetition of catastrophes in other instances. . . All 200 cases have in common the incident of illegitimacy, but it has almost 200 causes and these women's caliber and their problems make, of the 200, situations as various as one can believe any 200 cases could show. (Smith, 1934, p. 311)*

Nevertheless, through the 1930s, while illegitimate pregnancy frequently was thought to be the result of poor or inadequate social conditions or of feeble mindedness or other mental incapacity, social work writers often exhorted their colleagues to withhold approbation. Joanna Colcord (1923) asserted that, "In approaching unmarried maternity as social phenomenon, we want to get rid of the idea that unmarried mothers as a class differ especially from other girls of their age and status" (p. 171).

The attention of social caseworkers and casework writers was thus primarily on how to respond to the range of needs that unmarried mothers and their children had, rather than analyzing the "causes" of their undesirable situation.

The Racial Divide: Illegitimacy as Psychopathology Versus Culture

By the end of the 1940s and the 1950s, there was more systematic examination of the dynamics of illegitimacy. Although illegitimate births have always occurred among women of all classes and races in our society, there developed a marked difference in the theories explaining the same event among black and white women, with very little attention to women of other racial or ethnic groups. In identifying the modern foundation of social workers' responses to illegitimacy, Helen Harris Perlman summarized incisively this theoretical cleavage:

> *What do we believe—or know—to be the causes of sexual "acting out" that lead to unmarried motherhood? What motivates the individual girls or woman to violate what she "knows" (at least above the eyebrows) to be "wrong"? As soon as one examines the causation theory that has guided social work's practice with the girl and woman who is illegitimately pregnant, it becomes clear that something of a split or professional schizophrenia exists. Two different women are being talked about. One is white. The other black. And there are two different theoretical systems of causation. One is sociological and the other is psychoanalytic. The sociological is applied chiefly to Negro women; [sic] The psychoanalytic to white. (Perlman, 1964, p. 4)*

Practitioners and researchers generally assumed that out-of-wedlock childbearing among whites was the result of various types of individual psychopathology. In contrast, theories of "culture" or "social norms" were invoked to explain similar behaviors among minority, especially black women.

These two different explanations for illegitimate motherhood guided research about unmarried mothers and, by extension, professional social work practice. Thus, few researchers investigated either the psychological dimensions of early childbearing outside marriage among black women, or the social and cultural dimensions of the same among whites. There was some rational basis for the differing emphasis because childbearing outside of marriage historically has been more common among black than among white women. At the same time, the sharply differing approaches reflected a bias that severely limited our understanding of how complicated the multiple reasons are for early and out-of-wedlock pregnancy and childbearing among all young people.

Illegitimacy as Personal Pathology

I've thought about it a lot and I've only figured out one thing for certain. That the bunch of us in here got pregnant because we had some other big problem we just didn't know how to handle. All of us had a different problem, but one that had us pretty miserable. . .Of course I may be all wrong. (White teen mother in maternity home in 1960s)

As psychoanalysis took hold of social work in the 1940s, unmarried motherhood came to be defined explicitly as an expression of personal psychopathology among white women. Or, perhaps more accurately, the phenomenon among white women was considered more deviant relative to mainstream expectations, therefore of more professional and public concern:

In 1941 there was put forward the hypothesis that a cause-effect relationship exists between unresolved oedipal conflicts and unmarried motherhood. In the two decades that have followed a large number of writings by psychiatrists and social workers developed the themes of unconscious and unresolved emotional relationships with parents as the explanation for illegitimate pregnancy and unmarried motherhood. The assumptions made are that pregnancy and its culmination in unwed motherhood is a way of meeting a variety of unconscious (and sometimes preconscious) needs which include self-punishment for forbidden sex fantasies, punishment of one or both parents, self-assertion as a woman, self-assertion as a "whole" person, gratification of sexual fantasies in conjunction with or in competition with sexual parent figures, and so on. (Perlman, 1964, p. 288)

This theoretical orientation underlay practice literature in the area of services especially to adolescents and families. While social workers continued to focus their interventions on the disposition of the illegitimate child, they approached the problem with a more explicitly psychological perspective on the mother's motivations. Describing the consultative services provided to the venereal disease quarantine Isolation Hospital in Indianapolis by the Family Welfare Society, a caseworker explained the origin of the typical woman who had had sexual relations outside of marriage:

> *Patients are referred to the agency by the hospital in making suitable living arrangements or finding satisfactory employment for relief until wages are received, and for the help case work can give in working through personality problems of which the behavior is symptomatic. . .It is not surprising, then, to find that these girls feel the lack of a secure affectional relationship to parents and to other persons. . .In these cases the mother particularly seems to be a dominant, aggressive, unloving person. She is frequently rejecting and frankly punitive. (Little, 1944, p. 163)*

Frances Scherz (1947) of the Family Service Society in Atlanta warned her readers in the 1940s not to focus on the "emotional elements" precipitating unmarried motherhood to the exclusion of "sufficient recognition to environmental forces." Nevertheless, she recommended that caseworkers should attempt to "uncover and evaluate those emotional needs that are related to pregnancy and the coming decision [regarding whether or not to relinquish the infant]" (p. 58). This was because, "We know from psychiatric orientation and from casework experience that most unmarried pregnancy has a neurotic base. It is frequently a symptom of unresolved love–hate parental relationships, originating in early childhood" (p. 58).

Based on the assumption that "most unmarried mothers are serious neurotics" (Young, 1947, p. 28), social caseworkers focused on helping their clients identify the full range of motivations for conceiving outside of marriage so as to make a responsible—and conscious—decision about the child's future. Although social workers did not believe that it was their right to make such decisions for unmarried mothers, there was greater acceptance of more directive intervention to protect the illegitimate child from a neurotic mother's poor judgment. Leontine Young, one of the prominent writers on practice with unmarried mothers of the time, argued that social workers should be more "realistic" in assessing both the strengths and needs of young mothers and encourage them to make final decisions about relinquishing infants rather than support the then common solution of foster care. In describing the case of a young mother, she explained why good casework could include direct advice to permanently place a child:

> *In recognizing the girl's need for reassurance and permission, we solve also another question. Are we, in encouraging her to place the baby for adoption, in a psychological sense taking the baby away from her? We need to see that when the girl trusts us and is able to use our help she gives the baby to us. We do not take it from her. In essence the caseworker becomes a mother substitute, the good mother that the girl has been seeking, not the punitive mother she fears. And by giving the baby to us the girl can complete a drama of deep psychological meaning to her. (Young, 1947, p. 27)*

Scherz (1947) also explicitly advocated for the social worker to, "Take an active 'steering' role in helping the unmarried mother to make a good decision for herself and the child" (p. 57). Despite defining the process of "taking sides" on the issue of placing an illegitimate child as one that helps the client make the most reasoned decision, she concluded that, "...we are more 'on the side' of having the unmarried mother relinquish her baby. Our experience has shown that with rare exceptions, it is the more neurotic girl who keeps the child" (p. 61).

Such psychological assumptions about why unmarried women became pregnant, what influenced their decisions about the child's placement, and how social workers defined their objectives and methods with these clients must be viewed in the context of general social norms that, until quite recently, placed great stigma on pregnancy and childbearing outside of marriage. Even though the casework literature concerning unmarried motherhood throughout this century consistently referred to the impact of poverty, social disorganization, and other social and economic forces on women's choices about childbearing, there was a common belief that illegitimacy represented individual deviance and should be treated as such, albeit kindly and with sympathy.

The psychological studies conducted primarily by social workers and psychiatrists typically examined white unwed mothers from middle-class and working-class backgrounds. Samples tended to be drawn from social service settings such as homes for unmarried mothers and counseling agencies (Young, 1954). Studies employing primarily psychodynamic frameworks diagnosed and categorized the various forms of individual psychopathology that "drove" unmarried girls to have children. Young women suffering from a range of neurotic, borderline, and psychotic disorders were examined clinically to discover what sorts of disturbed family dynamics resulted in this characteristic acting-out behavior. Agency-based research using clients who sought (or whose families sought) professional assistance no doubt reinforced the assumption that illegitimate pregnancy was an expression of psychopathology.

By the mid-to-late 1960s, psychological studies were more methodologically sophisticated and often included control groups of nonparenting young women, providing a necessary comparative perspective that was based on stronger empirical evidence (Parker, 1969; Vincent, 1965). This later research found that, overall, there were fewer psychological differences between girls who became pregnant and girls in the general population than was asserted in the psychiatric literature.

While research using narrowly psychodynamic theory has not proven to be powerful in predicting which young women are more likely to become pregnant or young mothers, this does not mean that there are not significant psychological processes associated with heightened risk, as we will see in subsequent chapters. However, this earlier research did not adequately address some basic methodological problems such as whether observed psychopathology represented a pre-existing condition or resulted from the many stresses associated with being a young and single mother. This problem was especially difficult to disentangle empirically given the high degree of deviance that illegitimacy traditionally represented among the American white middle class. It is entirely possible that many of those pregnant young women who sought professional assistance with their situation from counseling and adoption agencies during the 1940s and 1950s today might choose a different course such as abortion or single motherhood without the presumed benefit of social services.

In addition to questions about its validity, early psychodynamic research too often asserted single-agent causality for behaviors that we now recognize to be multidetermined. The problem of conceptual singularity, however, is one that was shared by sociological and anthropological studies of illegitimacy among black and generally poor communities during the same time period to which we now turn.

Illegitimacy as Cultural Norm

With the first baby, it seemed pretty real to me, but I couldn't believe I was pregnant again. . .Like, I should have learned the first time. And then there were two more! But I don't love them any less because they're mistakes. . .There are a few things I hate about being a teenage mother, because there are people who think that we're doing it on purpose. At least I'm not. . .There are people who feel like it's really a big problem and it has to be stopped. I'm not saying it's not a problem. . .I don't expect you to say it's wonderful. I don't think it's wonderful. I wish I never had two kids. I faced reality. I wish I never had three kids. But still, you know, that doesn't make me terrible. I'm still human and I'm entitled to make say they're dumb mistakes, but still, that's how some things go. . .I want to pull myself up and change, you know, from where people are looking down on me. (16-year-old, low-income, black teenage mother, Chicago)

Until recently, virtually no major studies attempted to identify systematically the psychological dynamics of black teenagers who become pregnant and bear children. Rather, there is a well-developed tradition of social or cultural theories attempting to explain the higher incidence of out-of-wedlock births among black women. It is not clear why illegitimacy among minority groups has been treated mainly as a sociocultural phenomenon in contrast to the psychologically oriented research about whites' illegitimacy within the fields of psychiatry, psychology, and social work. Certainly, much higher rates of childbearing outside of marriage among black than among white women and their historically more accepting attitudes toward early and illegitimate childbearing (though perhaps less accepting and more resigned than some scholars and social workers assume) led to different explanatory models. Not only did this tendency reflect biases of researchers, but recent changes in patterns of sexual behavior and fertility especially among white young people require a more theoretically broad and even-handed approach to explaining contemporary adolescent parenthood. Nevertheless, the emphasis on cultural patterns and social factors under-lying the theoretically rich sociological and anthropological literature on illegitimacy provides an important foundation for our current understanding of social and cultural dimen-sions of teen pregnancy and parenthood, especially among the most economically disadvantaged who are at highest risk.

This body of sociocultural research on illegitimacy, drawn mainly from research in the United States, has been catego-rized usefully by social work scholar Robert Roberts (1966) according to a three-part typology: *cultural relativism, cultural absolutism, and cultural relationism.* Theories in each category focus on aspects of culture or subculture as the main set of variables explaining not only adolescent illegitimacy but also a range of behaviors that in some ways reflect the effects of class status on such important behaviors as sexual relations and family formation.

Cultural Relativism

According to Roberts' definition, the cultural relativists assume that,

> *Within complex societies such as the United States. . .sub-cultures exist which have norms about marriage and the family which are different from those held by the majority culture. They explain the higher illegitimacy rates of lower socio-economic classes and certain ethnic minorities on the basis that these groups hold counter-norms which either positively sanction unwed motherhood or treat it as a mor-ally neutral issue. (Roberts, 1966, p. 14)*

Three outstanding scholars in this tradition are E. Franklin Frazier, Kenneth Clark, and Lee Rainwater.

Frazier (1939), in his classic work, *The Negro Family in the United States,* asserted that migration from the rural south to the urban north had brought increasing disorganization to black families. He wrote:

> *The simple folkways of these peasant folk are conflict-ing more and more with the ideals and standards of the larger world as their isolation is being destroyed. More-over, the mobility of the population and the wider contacts are destroying the sympathetic relationships that were*

the bases of the old simple folkways. . .As the women in these rural communities move about and come into contact with the outside world, illegitimacy loses its harmless character in becoming divorced form the folkways of these simple peasants. It becomes part of the general disorganization of family life, in which the satisfaction of undisciplined impulses results in disease and in children who are unwanted and uncared for. (p. 99)

Frazier observed that as black migrants adjusted to the urban environment they developed a separate and self-reinforcing subculture of values that continued to encourage illegitimacy. He contrasted the patterns of poor blacks with those of middle-class black families in his controversial *The Black Bourgeoisie* (1957). There he described the black middle class as adopting an exaggerated version of mainstream norms and values in response to their economically, socially, and politically marginal position in a racist society.

Critical though he was of the "black bourgeosie," Frazier believed that illegitimate childbearing would decrease as blacks became more fully acculturated to northern city life. In this regard, the later works of writers such as Kenneth Clark describe patterns of family formation in urban ghettos that belie Frazier's optimistic predictions.

Thirty years after Frazier's influential work, Kenneth Clark wrote *Dark Ghetto* (1969). Writing from his experience as a psychologist working with youth in Harlem, Clark observed that middle-class and lower-class blacks held different attitudes toward sex that he thought explained the higher rates of illegitimacy among poor young women. He believed that among the middle class, sex is mainly symbolic and is used to attain status; for the poor, sex is an end in itself as it fulfills needs for affection and self-esteem. At the same time, sex among the poor carries with it no expectation of long-term obligation between partners. The birth of an illegitimate child also carries different meanings for poor women:

The innocent sophistication includes the total acceptance of a child if a child comes. In the ghetto, the meaning of the illegitimate child is not ultimate disgrace. There is not a demand for abortion or surrender of the child that one finds in more privileged communities. The child is proof of womanhood, something of her own to have. (Clark, 1969, p. 72)

Clark saw the ghetto as a seemingly insurmountable wall created by poverty and racism. His image of the bounded ghetto world was elaborated upon empirically and theoretically by sociologist Lee Rainwater. Based upon his research in the infamous St. Louis housing project, Puitt Igoe, Rainwater published *Behind Ghetto Walls* in 1970. Like Frazier and Clark, Rainwater observed a black lower-class subculture that included values and norms that were substantially different from those of middle-class society. He believed that one consequence of limited opportunity to move up and away from poverty is that the risks of unplanned pregnancy for adolescents are far outweighed by the immediate gratification of meeting needs for self-esteem and love provided by sexual relationships. In this cultural context, sex is a sign of maturity for girls, even in their early teens, and adolescent pregnancy does not threaten nonexistent prospects for future achievement.

In contrast to earlier writers, Rainwater asserted that even within a separate subculture, the poor simultaneously hold the same ideal norms and values as the middle class. Because the circumstances of poverty and racism militate against achieving these ideal standards, the poor develop an adaptive and more realistic set of alternative norms that guide daily living:

> *The study of lower-class subculture, lower-class styles of life, lower-class personalities, then, is the study of ways individuals and a class of people adapt to their disinheritances from their society. In their view, no valued, meaningful place is made for them, and they are denied the fundamental human equality that comes from having a functioning place in a society. Instead, they must find ways of living with the knowledge that they are an embarrassment in their world. (Rainwater, 1970, p. 373)*

In such a situation, Rainwater reasoned, bearing an illegitimate child at any age represents a rational decision, for at least some immediate emotional needs are met. The child is evidence to the young woman or man, of being a significant individual. Though a young woman may have no genuine expectation of recognition from the larger world, as she remains behind ghetto walls, her baby signals a transition from childhood to adulthood and is something of value in her world. This understanding of teen pregnancy as a means of meeting various needs that otherwise would not be met remains a recurring theme in contemporary understanding of teenage pregnancy and motherhood.

Little of theoretical significance in terms of sociocultural analysis has been written about illegitimacy among about whites. One interesting exception is Harry Caudill's (1963) history of eastern Kentucky, *Night Comes to the Cumberlands*, which portrays the roots and development of rural poverty in Appalachia. Caudill observed that certain customs that early immigrants brought to the area in combination with the ensuing poverty and physical isolation developed over time into a regional subculture that included high rates of teenage illegitimacy:

> *As hopelessness deepened general morality was undermined. . .They have taken a practical attitude toward sex and quite unashamedly behave as nature guides them. The illegitimate child—the mountaineer's terms is "base-born"—was never viewed with the disdain accorded such unfortunates in other societies. The bastards were altogether too numerous for such treatment to be practical. . .Having grown up without jobs of any kind or the worthwhile activities generally available to the nation's adolescent girls, they suffered from a nearly complete absence of the teachings and disciplines which instill pride in members of their sex. In short, their shabby environments and the loose standards of their families had made slatterns of them. (p. 289)*

These four writers, and others such as St. Clair Drake and Horace Cayton (1945), Oscar Lewis (1966), Elliot Liebow (1967), Carol Stack (1974), and Joyce Ladner (1971) share the assumption that nonmainstream behaviors such as out-of-wedlock pregnancy and childbearing represent patterned responses to an environment with few legitimate opportunities to meet individuals' needs. They view these patterned responses as logical means of adapting to harsh environmental conditions such as those in impoverished inner-city communities. What makes them "cultural" responses is that they develop an independent life of their own as they are taught to succeeding generations of children as long as environmental conditions remain the same. One of the enduring questions from this literature that occupies scholars and practitioners today is how fixed such patterns are if environmental conditions do change through for example, changes in social welfare policy or job opportunities. Current views about these issues will be addressed in the following chapter.

Cultural Absolutism

Diverging from culturally relativistic views of illegitimacy that recognize the functional meaning of subcultural adaptation is what Roberts termed *cultural absolutism*. According to this perspective, legitimacy is a universal, an absolute, norm, such as the incest taboo. There are no genuine counternorms, only breakdowns in normative functioning within a society. Unlike cultural relativists, who seek to understand the adaptive value of nonmainstream behaviors, cultural absolutists believe that the important question to answer is why certain individuals and groups fail to follow mainstream norms such as pregnancy and childbearing within marriage.

An early proponent of the absolutist positions was the anthropologist, Branislaw Malinowski. From his work with "savage" societies, Malinowski identified the "Principle of Legitimacy." In his essay, *Parenthood—the Basis of Social Structure,* he wrote, "To sum up, we have found that parenthood gives us the key to marriage, and that marriage is the key to a right understanding of sexual customs" (Malinowski, 1930, p. 41). In a published version of Malinowski's radio debates with writer Robert Briffault entitled *Marriage: Past and Present*, Malinowski (1956) asserted:

> *I believe that no human impulse is so deeply rooted as the maternal impulse in a woman; I believe that it is individual; and I believe that it is bound up with the institution of marriage. (p. 78)*

A later advocate of this view of the universality of the value of marital childbearing is William Goode. Goode (1961) used the notion of "anomie" to explain illegitimacy. Based on his research on Caribbean social structure, Goode described the inverse relationship between hierarchical location in the social stratum and deviation from mainstream norms. Trying to explain the high rates of illegitimacy he observed, Goode hypothesized that young women must make a "role bargain" with young men, risking pregnancy to gain a marriage partner. The need to do so is a function of social class: low social class in the Caribbean results in incomplete socialization to Western middle-class norms and values. Thus, as members of subcultures that experience poverty or racial exclusion achieve assimilation into the majority culture, with equal access to economic and social opportunities, the commitment to the principle of legitimacy increases. "The explanation for differing rates of illegitimacy is thus seen in relation to a breakdown in the socialization process for those groups with higher illegitimacy and not in the existence of counternorms" (Roberts, 1966, p. 16).

These two perspectives—cultural relativism and absolutism—offer quite different interpretations of adolescent illegitimacy. According to relativists, the higher incidence of out-of-wedlock childbearing and greater acceptance by poor black Americans is an expression of subcultural norms that have developed in response to environmental contingencies, especially poverty and racism. To label illegitimacy "deviant" is irrelevant in such a context, for it represents a logical adaptation to constrained social and economic conditions. The absolutist position views illegitimacy in terms of its departure from widely held mainstream norms about family formation—thought to be universally held—and as the result of distorted socialization.

Cultural Relationism

Roberts' third category of social theories of illegitimacy, *cultural relationism*, incorporates aspects of both relativistic and absolutist perspectives. He identifies the conceptual roots in sociologist Karl Mannheim's theory of knowledge:

> *Rejecting both the relativist and absolutist definitions of knowledge, Mannheim stated that "all of the elements in a given situation have reference to one another and derive their significance from this reciprocal relationship in a given frame of thought." (Roberts, 1966, p. 17)*

This middle position between the two theoretically (and sometimes ideologically) divergent views of illegitimacy represents a pragmatic melding that fits well with the cumulative weight of research findings. Social work scholar, Clark

Vincent (1961), employed this perspective in asserting that the principle of legitimacy is universally present as an ideal, but that specific cultural norms governing sexual behavior may vary both within and across societies. For example, norms concerning sexual activity have become significantly more permissive in the United States, even more so since Vincent wrote in 1961. Increased acceptance of nonmarital sexual activity has contributed to the increase in pregnancy and childbearing outside of marriage among white youth, while at the same time, there are conflicts among Americans about the appropriateness of such a change.

Hyman Rodman offered a particularly useful way of understanding what often appears to be a discrepancy between the stated mainstream values of many people and actual behavior that departs from such values. From his observations of lower-class families in Trinidad, Rodman (1971) described individuals' responses to an anomic situation in which one does not have available socially legitimate means to attain things that are legitimate to want, such as childbearing within marriage. He called this response *value stretch*:

> *By value stretch I mean that the lower-class person, without abandoning the general values of the society, develops an alternative set of values. Without abandoning the values of marriage and legitimate childbirth, he stretches these values so that a non-legal union and illegitimate children are also desirable. . .The result is that the members of the lower class in many areas have a wider range of values than others within a society. They share the general values of the society with members of other classes, but in addition they have stretched these values, or developed alternative values, which help them to adjust to their deprived circumstances. . .value stretch is an important response within the lower classes. (p. 195)*

Implicit in the notion of value stretch is that we may hold simultaneously more than one set, or even contradictory sets, of values. On the one hand, each society and its members have an identifiable core of ideals, or preferred values, and behaviors that may change over time but is evident in, for example, laws and policies governing conduct. The ongoing public policy and legal debates surrounding many aspects of sexuality including minors' access to contraception, abortion, and sexuality education reflect both our collective desire to regulate this aspect of our lives and the difficulty in reaching deep consensus on these profoundly important arenas. On the other hand, people must respond and adapt to many immediate environmental forces, drawing on their strengths to meet their immediate needs the best they can. These survival strategies may differ from ideal norms. Children, then, learn these strategies from their families and in their communities. In this way, cultural patterns develop over generations within subgroups that make up our heterogeneous society.

Many people living in extreme poverty over time are, in some respects, isolated economically, socially, politically, and psychologically from the central core of ideals of the larger society; yet, in daily life, they adapt to deprivation to survive. Thus, when marriage is not a likely prospect for young black— or white—women and men in impoverished communities, having children outside of marriage may be the only feasible way to form families. That does not mean that out-of-wedlock childbearing at any age is the preferred ideal. Rather, it may a realistic way to fulfill the normal human impulse to have children, or an unplanned consequence of sexual intimacy whose cost is worth the emotional gratification.

The continuing interest among social scientists in whether the high rates of out-of-wedlock childbearing among poor youth reflect genuinely alternative subcultural values is more than simply an academic debate. Social welfare programs and policies whose objectives include changing reproductive behavior and marital choices are based upon implicit, if not explicit, assumptions about the appropriate target for individual and environmental intervention, including values and, increasingly, attitudes. Indeed, federal social welfare policy encourages marriage as an explicit objective. Unfortunately, potentially productive discussion among practitioners and scholars about how patterns of behavior, such as how young men and women relate to one another and choose to form families in impoverished communities, often is sidetracked by mutual accusations of using the notion of a "culture of poverty" as a way to "blame victims" or of failing to hold young people responsible for their actions. Such simplistic views fail to recognize the deeply complex dynamics of how individuals are shaped both by immediate experiences and more distant social and cultural forces bearing historic and contemporary meaning. Rather than searching for the presence or absence of mainstream values, perhaps, it is more useful to examine which values and norms dominate in given situations and what influences them in those situations, along with the other many factors that motivate young people's sexual behavior and fertility.

Any analysis of childbearing outside of marriage among a particular subgroup, such as poor young people, must examine changes in the larger social context. How are we to understand the decline in marriage among childbearing teenagers when currently well over one third of all births in the United States are to unmarried women? In 1950, about 4% of all births were to unmarried women; by 2007, nearly 40% of births were outside of marriage. Another way of portraying this dramatic social change is in the comparison of nonmarital births among teenagers and to births among older women. In 1970, teenagers accounted for a little over half of births to unmarried women; in 2002, about one quarter of nonmarital births were to teenagers. It is thus critical to consider how, at the start of the new millennium, the relationship between marriage and parenthood have been transformed at least demographically; to what degree Furstenberg is justified in observing that perhaps teenagers were simply harbingers of more widespread changes in family formation (Furstenberg, 2008).

Summary

While recognizing the power of the social and cultural world as well as psychological dynamics that motivate individuals, we are wise to recall Helen Harris Perlman's observation that we are more than passive products of any singular force. Full recognition of the multiple forces in human development should lead to modest expectations about how well we can "explain," let alone predict any individual's action, especially through reductionistic perspectives:

> *No one of us can ever know the whole of another person, though we may sometimes delude ourselves to that effect. The reason for this lies not only in the subtle dimensions and interlacings of any personality but also in the shift and reorganization of new and old elements in the personality that take place continuously just because the person is alive*

in a live environment and is in interaction with it. Neverthe-
less, the person is a whole in any moment of his living. He
operates as a physical, psychological, social entity, whether
on the problems problem of his neurotic anxieties or of his
inadequate income; his is product-in-process, so to speak,
of his constitutional makeup, his physical and social envi-
ronment, his past experience, his present perceptions and
reactions, and even his future aspirations. It is this physical-
psychological-social–past-present-future configura-
tion that he brings to every life-situation he encounters.
(Perlman, 1957, p. 6)

We now turn to the current views on this configuration
and how we believe its constituent factors contribute to young
people's risk of early sex and its surrounding behaviors and
consequences.

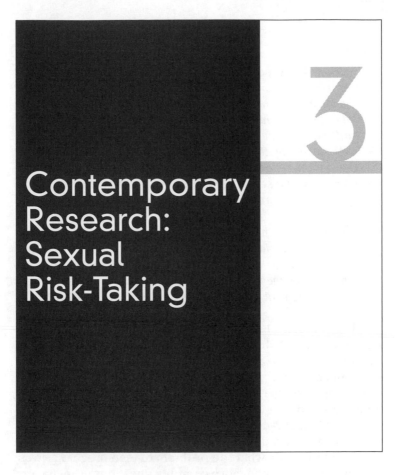

Contemporary Research: Sexual Risk-Taking

Beginning in the late 1960s, after the peak in modern rates of adolescent childbearing, teenage pregnancy became more narrowly defined as a social problem apart from the general issue of illegitimacy. There was a dramatic intensification of interest among researchers, social welfare practitioners, and members of the public in explaining and attempting to curb pregnancy among unmarried teenagers.

This shift in public perception required social workers and other social welfare professionals to reexamine their assumptions about unmarried mothers—who they were and what their needs were. The following frank admission by social group workers in 1971 describes the challenge.

> *Social workers are no strangers to uncertainty, particularly when they venture into new aspects of social problems or*

*work with new populations. What is striking about the work
with unmarried mothers is that, although it is an old problem,
the uncertainty has increased from decade to decade. In few
other instances have social workers felt the theoretical sands
shift beneath them to the extent that they have in the work
with unwed mothers. . .[in public and voluntary agencies]
the worker believes to some extent that she is confronted by
a client with a serious problem. What the problem consists
of and whose problem it is, however, she is not sure. . .For
the worker it is almost a relief to deal with the low-income
unmarried mother with her many problems in obtaining
concrete financial and related services. One then does not
have to face too quickly, or perhaps at all, the ambiguities
surrounding the treatment of unwed motherhood as a social
or psychological problem. (Kolodny & Reilly, 1972, p. 614)*

The theoretical sands surrounding practice with unmarried mothers did shift rapidly as traditional assumptions of
individual psychopathology and subcultural deviance were
challenged by new perspectives that defined pregnant and
parenting teenagers as a special population whose problems required innovative research and practice approaches
(Rains, 1971). Paradoxically, the "problematizing" of teenage
pregnancy occurred as nonmarital sex became more widely
acceptable. Exactly what the problem of teen pregnancy was,
and for whom, became more complex questions as teenagers
perceived a greater range of ostensibly appropriate choices
about their personal conduct, including sexual activity and
pregnancy resolutions (Lieberman, 1973).

Furstenberg (1976), whose landmark research on black
teen mothers in Baltimore remains one of the few longitudinal studies in the field, suggested four interrelated factors
accounting for the emergence of teen pregnancy as a serious
social problem. First, although fertility rates among adolescents had declined, the early mid-1960s saw a 25% increase
in the number of girls in their midteens in the population
and thus of potentially pregnant and parenting teenagers. Second, there was a general concern about population
growth that spurred "advocates of family planning to direct
their efforts toward specific groups within the population
that had experienced a high incidence of unintended and
unwanted births that might yield the largest payoff, given the
limited resources available" (Furstenberg, 1976, p. 9). Third,

teenagers having children were more likely than other women to be unmarried. In 1960, 15% of births to teens were out of wedlock; by 1970, the proportion had doubled. That is, the source of public concern was not primarily the absolute rate at which teenagers were giving birth, but rather the increasing ratio of births to teens who were not married, thus contributing to rising rates of illegitimacy (Furstenberg, 2008). Fourth, concern over teenage pregnancy developed hand-in-hand with vigorous efforts to reduce poverty. "Promiscuous sexual behavior, illegitimacy, and early marriage were singled out as cultural elements that contributed to the maintenance of poverty" (Furstenberg, 1976, p. 11). The growing public attention to teenage pregnancy prevention was motivated partly by the assumption that teenage motherhood was closely connected to various social and economic problems.

This assumption was supported by the weight of early research that suggested near universally dismal consequences of adolescent childbearing for all concerned. Current findings reveal much more diversity over the lives of young parents and their children than was previously reported, especially because more educational and other supports for teen parents are available. Still, in some respects, the outcomes are more negative and potentially long lasting among teens now who conceive and choose to parent. As rates of teen pregnancy among the general youth population have declined, those teenagers who become parents have become more concentrated among the most disadvantaged and vulnerable youth. Despite the overall decrease in adolescent pregnancy and childbearing, poor and minority youth continue to become adolescent parents at rates significantly above more affluent adolescents. Many of these most disadvantaged families now have reproduced multiple generations of unmarried adolescent mothers, and are passing on elevated risk for poor outcomes.

Another factor caused concern about teenage pregnancy during the 1960s and 1970s. As sexual mores became more liberal across society, sexual behavior of white and more affluent adolescents began to mirror that of poor and black youth who had higher rates of sexual activity, pregnancy, and nonmarital childbearing. The implicit assumption of earlier research that adolescents who conceived out of wedlock were, by definition, different from youth in the general population did not fit with the reality that unmarried girls and boys from various backgrounds and characteristics could, and did, engage in sexual activities, conceive, and get impregnated.

With major changes in patterns of sexuality and fertility, research about teen pregnancy has focused more closely on conceptually distinct and empirically observable antecedents to early sexual activity, patterns of contraceptive behavior, and pregnancy resolution among diverse youths. There are many strands of continuity from earlier psychological and anthropological or sociological research, but the knowledge base has expanded dramatically and incorporates important new elements. The early work of social work researchers such as Schinke (1978), Schinke et al. (1981), and others introduced a highly cognitive perspective on adolescent pregnancy prevention, emphasizing life skills and relationship training, influencing strongly the direction of prevention services (Cobliner, 1974).

Today, most explanatory models no longer link motivation for early sexual initiation directly to unmarried motherhood (Zelnick & Kanter, 1977; Gordon, 1996). Instead, each decision—whether, when, how often, and with whom to have coitus; whether to use birth control at any given time; whether to have an abortion or to carry a pregnancy to term; whether to keep or give up a child for adoption; and finally whether to marry or remain single—is regarded as a discrete act that is multidetermined and potentially independent. The dominant explanations that inform practice are not generalized theories of adolescent illegitimacy per se; rather, they are efforts to account for different levels of adolescents' sexual risk-taking behaviors that can result in pregnancy, having a child, or increasing concern about the possibility of contracting a sexually transmitted illness (STI) (Shah & Zelnick, 1981). In other words, we no longer ask why, in a global sense, youth go astray, but why they make poor specific choices.

Despite—or perhaps as evidence of—the overall trend toward freer individual choice, not all adolescents engage in sexual intercourse; those teens who are sexually active do not all face the same risk of pregnancy and STI; and those teens who become pregnant do not all become unmarried mothers. Different degrees of risk of each of these events are associated with adolescents' emotional, social, and economic characteristics as well as common developmental features that often transcend their socioeconomic status and community characteristics. At the same time, although discernible patterns of risk are clear, none determines any particular outcome. That is because, as Mary Frances Smith correctly observed about unmarried mothers in 1934, each woman is motivated by a unique combination of factors as, of course, are their male partners.

Sexual Risk-Taking: Common Factors

"I got married at 16 to get away from my family and had a baby. I went from an alcoholic abusive father (who never worked) to an alcoholic abusive husband (who didn't work)." Terry, a white single mother of three, divorced her husband when the abuse and lack of money became intolerable. She recently completed her GED and began a job as a nurse's aid. Terry lives in a small southeastern city with her boyfriend, Jack, their young daughter, and her two children from her previous marriage. They recently faced eviction and home-lessness because both she and her boyfriend lost their jobs. Terry hopes to go to technical college in the future, but in addition to her financial difficulties, she has her hands full with a toddler, a son with severe Tourette syndrome, and another son whose behavior is uncontrollable at home. With little education, a poor local economy, and similarly poor relatives, their financial situation continues to be extremely tenuous, despite their hard work and aspirations. The psychosocial difficulties of her youth set the stage for long-term vulnerability to poverty and its attending stresses.

Adolescents like Terry are among those at high risk of becoming pregnant and single parents with poor prospects of a significantly more secure future. As a group, they share certain aspects of their individual, family, peer, and community environments. Some youths possess many of these characteristics, spanning multiple domains of their environment, others few. Some characteristics appear to be related to only a few of the high-risk choices, others to all of them. In general, the more of these factors present in a young person's life, the higher the risk of becoming an adolescent parent; conversely, the more protective factors a teen possesses, the lesser the chances of early pregnancy and parenthood.

There is a considerable body of empirical studies identifying what factors are most closely associated with high-risk sexual behaviors and childbearing and what factors can diminish those risks. Their findings support various theories rather than pointing to clear and neat explanations for all young people. Together they provide a strong basis for differential risk assessment of early and unprotected sex among diverse young men and women.

Overall, poverty is the strongest single factor associated with teenage pregnancy and childbearing because so many threats to optimal development converge to decrease young persons' motivation and ability to avoid early parenthood. Yet, young people who are not poor also engage in activities that result in early childbearing and share individual characteristics of those at highest risk. The risk of having early and unprotected sex, and thus of pregnancy and STI, is increasingly conceptualized as an integral aspect of the overall risk of other high-risk activities that threaten a young person's physical and emotional healthy development.

Social workers typically assess clients in terms of history and current functioning across multiple individual and environmental domains such as the family system, peer, and other relationships. This organizing framework guides the following review of the most recent and reliable research findings on antecedents to high-risk teenage sexual behavior and childbearing. Arranged by Kirby (2007), according to their conceptual similarity and interrelationships, these clusters of antecedent factors are grouped here by their environmental level. Although we focus here on describing antecedents to sexual activity, the following chapter will synthesize the major findings in terms of their contribution to a continuum of high-risk behavior.

Individual Characteristics

Biological Antecedents Specific biological characteristics such as level of testosterone, age of menarche, overall physical development that signal early maturity are risk factors for early sexual initiation (Zabin & Hayward, 1993; Miller, 1998). Initiating sexual activity early heightens risk of pregnancy partly because typical aspects of normal cognitive and emotional development often reduce younger teens' capacity to use birth control effectively. Younger teens are more likely to use condoms, while older teens prefer to use contraceptive pills or Depo Provera. However, although the longer-lasting medical contraception protects effectively against pregnancy, condoms protect most effectively against both pregnancy and STIs.

Chronological age per se is a risk factor for sexual activity, pregnancy, and STI. As teens get older, they are more likely to have sexual intercourse and to have increasing numbers of partners. Some of the social effects of age that act to increase sexual risks include intensifying pressure from peers, perceived norms favoring sexual activity, and more opportunities to have sex that often come with greater independence from adult supervision. Within this developmental context, however, girls and boys face somewhat different risks. Boys report having more partners and also using condoms more regularly, whereas girls contract STIs more frequently (Kirby, 2007).

Attachment to and Success in School One of the most troubling correlates of teen parenthood is abridged educational attainment with its impact on future economic achievement. Earlier research assumed that pregnancy or childbirth were usually direct causes of teenagers dropping out of school. Although this is certainly true for some young people, school problems and failure precede pregnancy for many adolescents. Adler observes that, ". . .those teens who are already doing poorly in school, have low self-esteem, and do not see much chance of gaining esteem through academic performance appear to see pregnancy and motherhood as an alternative path" (Becker, Rankin, & Rickel, 1998, p. 69).

Thus, poor attachment to and performance in school are highly significant risk factors for early sexual initiation, pregnancy, and childbearing (Resnick et al., 1997; Darroch, Landry, & Oslak, 1999). Common indicators include educational achievement such as grades and promotion, a sense of connectedness to school, valuing education, and educational aspirations (Ohannessian & Crockett, 1993; DiBlasio & Benda, 1990; Resnick, et al, 1997; Halpern, Joyner, Udry, & Suchindran, et al., 2000; Lammers et al., 2000; Raine et al., 1999). Kirby (2007) reports that active involvement in school organizations, for example school-based religious organizations among white teens and clubs among African American teens, reduces the risk of pregnancy.

In some instances, students who perform poorly academically and become pregnant may have undiagnosed learning disabilities (Iversen & Farber, 1999). In the context of chaotic and understaffed public schools in poor communities, children often receive inadequate individual attention to identify the presence of such problems or to provide effective remedial services.

A few studies of schools find that characteristics such as income level, ethnicity, and levels of vandalism by students act as risk factors for pregnancy (Kirby, 2001). However, insofar as the students come from poor neighborhoods, it is difficult to separate the impact of the school from that of its surrounding community.

Attachment to Religious Institutions The impact of religion on adolescents' sexuality is a complicated issue (Benda, 2002). Youths who attend religious institutions are less likely to initiate sex and have fewer partners when sexually active (Brewster et al., 1998; Seidman, Mosher, & Aral, 1994). The direction of influence between religions affiliation and sexual activity is not clear; it may be that teens whose sexual behavior violates their religious tenets do not feel comfortable attending religious activities (Kirby, 2007).

At the same time, some research finds that greater religiosity is related to less use of contraception when teens do have intercourse (Kirby, 2001). It is not surprising that being more religious might decrease rather than increase sexually active teens' effective use of contraception. Many young people are deeply ambivalent about having sex. They often feel conflicted or guilty about being sexually intimate, because it contradicts their or their parents' religious beliefs and values. These young men and women may express their ambivalence by not taking the positive steps to prevent pregnancy that would require open acknowledgment of their actions.

Teenagers' Own Sexual Beliefs, Attitudes, and Skills This category of factors is widely viewed by researchers as one of the most potent antecedents to sexual decision making and also constitutes the most theoretically specific and coherent basis for intervention currently used to reduce high-risk sexual behavior. Perhaps the most common practice approaches among programs to reduce risk of early and unprotected sex to avoid STIs and pregnancy focus on changing youths' attitudes, intentions, and capacity to act in accordance with those intentions. The widely influential "Theory of Reasoned Action" assumes that among these individual level factors, the most predictive of actual behavior is the "person's intention to perform that behavior" (Fishbein, 1997, p. 81). Guilamo-Ramos, Jaccard, Dittus, Gonzalez, and Bouris (2008) elaborate this theory and include social learning concepts in their framework that predicts intentions of high-risk youth to have sex. The model assumes that "for an intention to become a behavior, the adolescent must have the necessary knowledge and skills to perform the behavior; face no environmental constraints on performing the behavior; find the behavior salient, personally meaningful, or important; and be able to manage habitual and automatic processes" (Fishbein, 2000; Guilamo-Ramos et al., 2008, p. 30).

Several factors influence the development of a behavioral intention. First are the expectancies associated with the behavior; that is, how positive or negative are the anticipated consequences associated with the behavior. For example, many low-income African American young women believe that certain medical forms of contraception, such as the pill, often cause serious illness (Witte, 1997). Although some women do experience annoying side effects, this exaggerated view contributes to many sexually active young women choosing the risks of unprotected sex over birth control. The same decision to have unprotected sex may, paradoxically, result from young persons who believe that no form of birth control can effectively prevent conception when they decide to have intercourse in response to many complex motivations.

Second are social norms that can act as pressure to perform—or avoid—a particular behavior. Guilamo-Ramos et al. (2008) distinguish between "injunctive" and "descriptive" norms (p. 31). Injunctive norms are those that reflect behavioral approval or disapproval by people with whom young people are motivated to comply. Parents may attempt to inculcate norms that include disapproval of having sex before marriage, although peers having sex models a conflicting norm. Descriptive norms refer to perceptions of peers' behavior that may or may not be accurate. Studies of sexual activity among adolescents regularly reveal that they overestimate the number of their peers who are having sex. Such disparity between perceived norms of behavior and actual behavior among peers can lead teens to have a false sense of what is normative and thus inadvertently reinforce their choice to engage in risky behavior.

The third factor that influences behavioral intention is self-efficacy, or how confident an individual is that he or she can be successful in carrying out the behavior. If a young woman has the intention of not engaging in sexual intercourse, she will be more likely to remain abstinent if she feels confident that her "refusal" skills will enable her to avoid having sex; or if she wishes to protect herself from conceiving and contracting an STI, she will be more likely to attempt to use a condom if she believes she is capable of gaining her partner's agreement and using the condom effectively.

Fourth is self-image, which is especially important for adolescents because part of their identity development includes defining and identifying with others who represent a valued image. In an effort to present themselves in a socially approved manner, young people tend to behave in some ways that are similar to those whose images are considered to be positive in their milieu.

Current findings consistent with this general theoretical framework suggest the following summary of significant influences on teens' sexual activity and contraceptive choices (Kirby, 2007, p. 66):

- Teens are more likely to have sex, to have sex more frequently, and to have more partners if they have permissive attitudes toward premarital sex.
- Teens are less likely to have sex if they have taken a virginity pledge.
- Sexually active teens are more likely to use birth control if:
  - they believe that boys share responsibility for pregnancy prevention;
  - they believe that condoms do not reduce sexual pleasure;
  - they believe that their partner will appreciate their using a condom;
  - they have positive attitudes toward condoms and other forms of birth control;
  - they perceive more benefits and fewer costs and barriers in using condoms;
  - they have greater confidence in their ability to demand condoms and other forms of birth control;
  - they have greater confidence in their ability to use condoms and other forms of birth control;
  - they have greater motivation to use condoms or other forms of birth control to avoid pregnancy and STD or HIV;
  - they intend to use condoms;
  - they carry condoms with them.

In chapter 5, we will discuss how these particular influences on sexual decision making inform pregnancy prevention programs.

Personality Factors: Patterns of High-Risk Behavior and Emotional Distress Adolescents are at high risk for pregnancy and childbearing if they engage in what are considered to be "problem" behaviors such as use of alcohol or drugs, delinquency, or running away. In particular, alcohol and drug use are two high-risk behaviors that are associated with teens engaging in early, unprotected sex, having sex more often and with more partners, and pregnancy. However, the association is not uniformly supported by all studies, nor is it known whether there is a causal relationship between substance use and high-risk sexual behavior, and if there is a causal relationship, what direction might it be. One plausible theory is that these particular behaviors may be part of teens' general risk-taking dispositions. If so, it is important to understand better what increases youths' proclivity for sensation seeking and other motivations for behaviors that may threaten their safety and well-being. The other common assumption is that drug and alcohol use diminishes both inhibitions and rational decision making, resulting in riskier sexual behavior. Although this assumption may be regarded as almost conventional wisdom, there is not sufficient empirical evidence to conclude that chemically-induced disinhibition directly influences teenagers' sexual decision making.

These findings, albeit tentative, emerge from an abundant body of psychological research examining adolescents' sexual activity as part of a pattern of high-risk behaviors that are not considered to be appropriate for their healthy development. In spite of the recent changes in what is widely considered to be normative for adolescents, current research continues to find an association between early sexual activity, unprotected sex, pregnancy, and STI with other high-risk behavior that compromises adolescents' physical and mental health.

These high-risk behaviors overlap with another subset of risk factors related to mental health. Adolescents who experience high levels of stress, depression, suicidal ideation and attempts, and other psychiatric conditions as well as fear of untimely death are more likely to be sexually active (Kirby, 2007, p. 66; Bower, 1997, p. 229). The presence of these factors increases the risk of all sexual and reproductive decisions leading to childbearing among teenagers. Regarding substance use, we do not know the direction of causation, or whether they co-occur within a generally stressful and negative environment.

Although not all high-risk behavior is an indication of a mental health problem, there is some evidence that pregnant and parenting teens are more emotionally troubled than other young women. For example, Thomas and Rickel (1995) found that Minnesota Multiphasic Personality Inventory (MMPI) scores of pregnant or parenting teens revealed more "maladjustment" than those of their high school peers. Becker et al. (1998) suggest that these MMPI profiles reflect "symptoms of trauma" in adolescents whose early pregnancies are aspects of intergenerational dysfunction (p. 67). In their comparison of adolescents who anticipate being sexually active within 6 months with those who do not expect to have sex, Whitaker, Miller, and Clark (2000) found significant differences in measures of psychological health. So-called anticipators reported more heavy alcohol use, marijuana use, lower self-esteem, less controls among women, and more hopelessness (p. 114). Despite a relative dearth of information about how particular psychological dysfunction influences sexuality, there is compelling evidence that teens with mental health problems are at greater risk for both sexual and other nonsexual behaviors that may compromise their well-being.

Among practitioners, there appears to be widespread belief that low self-esteem contributes significantly to various poor outcomes. However, there is mixed evidence regarding how self-esteem operates as either protective or risk factor for high-risk sexual behavior. Kirby (2007) summarizes this inconclusive literature:

> *A few studies, including some with large samples that are representative of teens across the United States, have found that self-esteem and positive self-concept are protective factors against initiation of sex, use of contraception, and pregnancy. However, the large majority of studies has found that self-esteem and self-concept are not significantly related to sexual behavior. A few studies have found self-esteem to be protective only for girls or only for middle school (as opposed to high school) students. At least one study actually found that having sex can increase self-esteem. Thus,*

the relationships between these factors and sexual behavior are unclear and probably quite complex. (p. 66)

These findings are extremely important to consider for planning interventions to decrease sexual risk-taking. Although few would deny that, on balance, high self-esteem is in itself a desirable attribute for optimal psychosocial development, the research should caution against using higher self-esteem as an adequate independent outcome for prevention programs.

Participation in athletics There is a small set of findings that suggest that girls who participate in sports tend to delay sexual initiation, have sex less frequently and with fewer partners, use contraception more frequently, and are less likely to become pregnant than female nonathletes (Kirby, 2007; Sabo et al., 1999). In contrast, athletic participation does not appear to act as a protection against high-risk sexual behavior for boys. However, the nature of this relationship is unclear, as female athletes also tend to engage less in other risky behaviors. Thus, it is difficult to know how sports participation influences girls' sexual decision making independent of other risk factors.

Family Environment

The family is usually the most immediate and encompassing of socioemotional environments for young people. Youths at greatest risk of early pregnancy and parenthood come from poor families that live in impoverished communities. However, particular characteristics of family structure and process contribute to children's level of high-risk sexual behavior regardless of socioeconomic status (Corcoran 2000).

Family Structure and Economic Status The overall risk of adolescent girls conceiving and of boys impregnating a girl is higher in single-parent families, whether the parents have been divorced, separated, or were never married (Inazu & Fox, 1980; Rodgers, 1999; Hogan & Kitagawa, 1985; Newcomer & Udry, 1987; Forste & Heaton, 1988; Ku, Sonenstein, & Pleck, 1993; Lauritsen, 1994; Moore, Morrison, and Glei, 1995; Pick & Palos, 1995; Dorius & Barber, 1998). Until recently, researchers believed that lower income among single-mother families was the primary source of risk of teen pregnancy and other negative child outcomes (McLanahan and Sandefur, 1994). Current research suggests that the significance of family structure is more complicated. Some research suggests that living without two married parents may exert independent effects on children's development, including sexual behavior (Afxentiou & Hawley, 1997; Upchurch, et al, 1998). That is, all other things being equal, the most protective family context for young people is living with married biological parents (Kirby, 2007).

Moore and Chase-Lansdale (1999) suggest three major theories of the impact of family structure on teens' risk of early sex and pregnancy. The "socialization hypotheses" assert that parents "socialize their children for appropriate sexual behavior through norms they teach and by acting as roles of marital or non-marital sexual behavior" (p. 4). Supervision and monitoring hypotheses suggest that the level of parental supervision directly influences adolescents' sexual activity; that in two-parent homes, children simply have less opportunity to have sex than when only one parent is available. Third, the marital transition hypotheses assume that when single-parent families are formed through marital disruption, children respond to the family instability by assuming adult roles early, such as that of mother. No existing research definitively favors any of these theories. From the perspective of family systems, they are certainly not mutually exclusive and each can reasonably affect an individual young person over the course of adolescence.

In terms of other significant family demographic characteristics, teens are more likely to have sex early, become pregnant, and give birth when parents have low levels of education, low income, and received welfare for more than one generation (Zelnick, Kantner, & Ford, 1981; Hogan & Kitagawa, 1985; Forste & Heaton, 1988; Grady, Hayward, & Billy, 1989; Brewster, 1994; Afxentiou & Hawley, 1997; Roosa, Tein, Reinholtz, & Angelini, 1997; Upchurch et al, 1999). Risk is also heightened when adolescents' own unmarried mothers are dating and sexually active, and when mothers or older sisters give birth as adolescents (East, Felice, & Morgan, 1993; East, 1996; East & Shi, 1997; Widmer, 1997; Kirby, 2007).

Of course, not all families that are poor or that live in impoverished communities have characteristics associated with greater risk of teen pregnancy and childbearing. There is great diversity among poor families and within the most distressed communities. Moore and Chase-Lansdale (1999) report that within poor, predominantly African American urban communities, the age at which adolescent girls become sexually active varies according to the strength of the relationship with their parents. Adolescents' perceptions of support and cohesion among neighborhood adults also lower their risk of early pregnancy (Moore & Chase-Lansdale, 1999).

We also know that individual resilience and other strengths help people survive—even flourish—in deeply nonnurturing circumstances (Saleeaby, 1997; Iversen & Farber, 2000). Despite the diversity among families within impoverished communities, the profound challenges of being poor can make it difficult for parents to provide children with the emotional and material resources necessary to reach their individual potential as well-functioning adults (Brooks-Gunn, Duncan, Klebanov, & Sealand, 1993). Zabin and Hayward (1993) suggest how family life can be affected by poverty in inner-city communities:

> Normally, however, even though the individual increasingly differentiates him or herself as an independent person, the family remains an important influence throughout adolescence. This pattern—the gradual intrusion of broader influences to the sphere of a strong and sustained family—is less common in areas of urban poverty. In these areas, few families are intact, and single mothers must often struggle to provide basic necessities for their children. Subject to the multiple stresses of poverty and deprivation, often tied to low-paying jobs with difficult hours, parents may have little time and energy for children. Inevitably, children are often without supervision, and the overall influence of family life is diminished. (p. 48)

Family Dynamics, Attachment and Communication Certain family processes also appear to shape an adolescent's sexual behavior and subsequent fertility outcomes (Farber & Iversen, 1998). The significance of the general familial environment is apparent in research that finds young people who have lived either in foster care or kinship care at significantly elevated risk for high-risk reproductive behavior (Carpenter et al., 2001). Youth in foster care become sexually active an average of 7.2 months and those in kinship care 12 months earlier than their peers; youths in both circumstances of care first conceive almost a year before other girls (Carpenter et al., 2001). Yet, beyond the basic assumption that families act as environmental constraints to risky choices, the current research on how families influence teenagers' sexual behavior reveals little consistency or clear empirical basis to direct prevention practice.

A recent review of theory-based studies of predictors of adolescent sexual behavior and intention found that, "the environmental constraint exhibiting the strongest variability in findings was parental monitoring/supervision" (Buhi & Goodson, 2007, p. 8). On the one hand, according to some research, less monitoring and supervision by parents is related to earlier initiation of sex especially among boys, greater frequency of sex and unprotected sex, with more partners (Miller, Forehand, & Kitchick, et al., 2000; Romer, Stanton, Galbraith, Feigelman, Black, and Li, 1999; DiClemente et al., 2001; Huebner and Howell, 2003; Li, Feigelman, & Stanton, 2000; Unger, Molina, & Teran, 2000; Longmore, Manning & Giordano, 2001). Some studies find that adult supervision such as setting guidelines for completing schoolwork, curfews, recreational activities, can decrease teenagers' sexual risk-taking (Ku et al, 1993; Benda & DiBlasio; Hovel, Sipan, Blumbert, Atkins, Hofstetter, & Kreitner, 1994; Luster & Small, 1994; Small & Luster, 1994; Danziger, 1995; Luster & Small, 1997; Upchurch et al., 1998). When teens spend more time home alone or with a peer of the opposite sex without a parent present, they are more likely to have sex (Dilorio et al., 2004; Perkins, Luster, Villarruel, & Small, 1998). In a study of Black and Hispanic families, Miller et al. (1999) found that parental monitoring, especially by the mother, is strongly associated with teenagers having less frequent intercourse and fewer sexual partners.

On the other hand, many studies find no empirical relationship between monitoring and the same outcomes (Buhi and Goodson, 2007), and there is a small body of research that finds only indirect effects of parental supervision.

It is likely that one source of the conflicting findings is methodological inconsistency, that is, in what is being measured and how. In addition, there are complexities in processes of parental monitoring that are not always captured across studies. For example, supervision that is too restrictive can backfire and result in teenagers defying parents' rules, especially if mothers are psychologically intrusive (Dorius & Barber, 1998). In other words, either too much or too little supervision can contribute to an adolescent's tendency to begin to have sex early. Although there is no magic line dividing adequate from overly strict supervision, adolescents need to know that their parents or guardians care about their well-being enough to have clear expectations for their behavior.

As a general rule, strong emotional attachment to parents who closely monitor their children can protect them from the destructive impact of dangerous neighborhoods, peers, or other threats to well-being (Kirby, 2007). Yet, much else remains unknown about the nature of family influence on adolescents' sexual development.

For example, there is no consensus about the impact of either the quality or quantity of parent–child communication on youths' sexual activity. Some studies found that open communication about sexuality-related issues decreases teens' early sexual debut, frequency of sex, and unprotected intercourse (Moore, et al, 1986; Fisher, 1989; East, 1996; Miller et al, 1998). Other research finds mixed impact or no effect on adolescents' sexual activity (Inazu & Fox, 1980; Thomson, 1982; Cvetkovich & Grote, 1983; Fisher, 1989; Casper, 1990; Christopher et al, 1993; Hovell et al., 1994; Widmer, 1997). The protective impact of open communication about sexuality is most apparent for mothers and daughters (Kirby, 2007). When teens and parents feel strongly connected, positive communication has a stronger influence on teens' sexual behavior. In particular, spending more time with mothers is associated with later initiation of sexual activity. However, it appears that the strength of the influence of familial closeness is stronger for girls than for boys (Ramirez-Valles et al., 2002; Ream & Savin-Williams, 2005; Davis & Friel, 2001; Rose et al., 2005).

Firm conclusions about how intrafamilial communication influences children's sexual activity are especially difficult to draw because of the methodological limitations mentioned earlier. Studies use different measurements of communication and different samples. So findings often are not comparable on many dimensions or across racial and ethnic groups. Overall, however, recent evidence affirms that when parents initiate conversation about sexuality-related topics before children are sexually active, greater communication contributes to reducing sexual risk-taking (Kirby, 2007).

In terms of the content of communication, the weight of research finds that parents' attitudes toward and values about premarital sex have a notable impact on their children's sexual behavior. Conservative parental values about teen and premarital sex discourage children from becoming sexually active and contribute to less frequent sexual intercourse and fewer sexual partners (Baker, Thalberg, & Morrison, 1988; Weinstein & Thornton, 1989; Jaccard & Dittus, 1991; Hovell et al., 1094; Small & Luster, 1994; Jaccard, Dittus, & Gordon, 1996; Luster & Small, 1997; Resnick et al., 1997; Widmer, 1997; Buhi, 2007; Kirkby, 2007). At the same time, sexually active adolescents whose parents express positive attitudes toward contraception use birth control more effectively (Jorgensen & Sonstengard, 1984; White, 1987). Conversely, when parents express more permissive attitudes about teen and premarital sex and less positive attitudes about contraception, children are more likely to be sexually active earlier, have sex more often and without birth control, conceive and become teen parents (Kirby, 2007).

We cannot specify in detail the types or content of family communication that influence teenagers' sexual behavior. Nevertheless, there is compelling evidence that when children feel emotionally close to their parents, and parents consistently supervise their activities in developmentally appropriate ways and express strong preference for sexual abstinence, young people are more likely to delay having sex and to use birth control if they do have intercourse. Despite the many competing forces in the complex environments of adolescents today, parents can exert considerable influence toward helping their teenagers avoid early sex and pregnancy through nurturing an emotionally warm environment in which children have clear understanding of parents' expectations for their behavior inside and outside of their home.

Child Sexual Abuse There is strong growing evidence of a relationship between child abuse, particularly sexual abuse, and teen pregnancy. Sexually victimized children have earlier sexual debuts as teenagers, more sexual partners, use birth control less, and are more likely to become pregnant or impregnate a girl (Boyer & Fine, 1992; Butler Burton, 1992; Luster & Small, 1994; Small & Luster, 1994; Miller et al, 1995; Nagy, DiClimente, & Adcock, 1995; Browining & Laumann,

1997; Luster & Small, 1997; Roosa et al., 1997; Stock, Bell, Boyer, & Connell, 1997; Kirby, 2007).

We do not yet understand the mechanism of impact of sexual abuse and other forms of child maltreatment on girls' psychosexual development. Developmental psychologist Musick (1993) suggests that" for a sizable group of adolescent mothers, contemporary social and sexual relationships with males may be reenactments of patterns established earlier in life: lessons of victimization learned all to well" (p. 91). Extending this analysis, Becker et al. (1998) suggest that early child abuse often results in specific psychopathological conditions that mediate later high-risk behaviors, including early and unprotected sexual activity. In particular, they identify dissociation, depression, and borderline personality disorder as conditions that increase the likelihood of young women being revictimized sexually. We know even less about the effect of child maltreatment on boys, although there is some evidence that experiencing physical abuse, sexual abuse, and/or having a mother who was battered increases the likelihood of boys impregnating an adolescent girl (Anda et al., 2001).

Peer Environment

Peer Attitudes and Behavior Adolescents are influenced both by what their peers are actually doing and by their perceptions of what their peers are doing. These perceptions of peers' attitudes and actions affect teens' own intentions regarding sexual behavior as well as their actual choices about whether to have sex and whether or not to use birth control if they are sexually active (Buhi, 2007; Bearman, Bruckner, Brown, Theobald, & Philliber, 1999; Kirby, 2007).

Both teenage boys and girls are more likely to initiate sexual activity when they are popular with peers who are older, sexually active, and hold permissive attitudes toward premarital sex (Alexander & Hickner, 1997; Benda & DiBlasio, 1991; Whitaker & Miller, 2000; Carvajal, Parcel, Basen-Engquisit, Banspach, Coyle, and Kirby 1999; Gibson & Kempf, 1990; Bearman & Bruckner, 1999; Kirby, 2007). Being popular and socially active with peers also heightens chances of early sexual activity (Kirby, 2001). Conversely, adolescents whose peers have less permissive attitudes report less intention to initiate sexual activity and are more likely to remain abstinent (Watts & Nagy, 2000; O'Sullivan & Brooks-Gunn, 2005).

Once they become sexually active, young men and women are less likely to use birth control if their peers use drugs or alcohol, and if they do not support use of contraception (Boyer, Tschann, & Shafer, 1999; DiClemente et al, 1996; Whitaker & Miller, 2000). Overall, the risk of childbearing is increased when a best friend has been pregnant (Holden et al., 1993). Being perceived by peers as an aggressive child and gang membership increase sexual risk-taking as well (Underwood, Kupersmidt, & Coie, 1996; Thornberry, Smith, & Howard, 1997; Kirby, 2007).

It is not surprising that associating with others who engage in risky behavior can encourage a youth to do likewise, but the direction of influence is not clear. Do young men and women who are predisposed to high-risk behavior seek like-minded friends? Or do young people engage in high-risk behavior and then find peers to whom they are similar? Contrary to traditional conventional wisdom, recent research on peer culture suggests that young people are influenced more strongly by their families than by their friends. Nevertheless, if families are not available or are not actively involved in their children's daily lives, the potential for "outside" influences grows.

Partner Characteristics and Relationships The impact of a young person's partner on his or her sexual behavior occurs in complex ways. Unlike other significant antecedent factors such as poverty, family structure, or substance use that increase the risk of all sexual behaviors related to childbearing, intimate partnerships can affect sexual outcomes in different ways.

Young women and men are more likely to initiate sexual activity, including intercourse, when they are "going steady" in an ongoing and close relationship, if they are having sex with more than one partner, or when the man is older than the woman (Blum, Buehring, & Rinehart, 2000; Halpern, Joyner, Udry, & Suchindran, 2000; Marin et al., 2000). However, steady sexual partners are also much more likely than other couples to use birth control effectively (Kastner, 1984; Weisman, Plichta, Nathanson, Chase, Ensminger, & Robinson, 1991) and so avert pregnancy. Partners who discuss HIV and other STIs and methods of contraception are openly more likely to use condoms and to practice birth control.

When a young woman or man is in a relationship that includes sexual pressure, coercion, or abuse, sexual initiation occurs earlier, intercourse is more frequent, and contraception is used less frequently (Kirby, 2001). The significance of early sexual abuse was mentioned above in the context of the family. When a young person has been victimized by sexual abuse, she or he remains more vulnerable to engaging in unwanted sexual activity.

There are particular risks for young women, especially in middle school, when they have partners who are 3 or more years older (Kirby, 2007). They are more likely to initiate sexual activity, less likely to use contraception, and more likely to contract an STI. The risk of STI is especially acute when the older partner has or has had multiple sexual partners.

Early sexual activity brings multiple and serious risks. Teens who start having sex early are less likely to use birth control, and thus more likely to conceive and become a parent. They also tend to have more lifetime sexual partners and are less likely to use condoms. These two factors—the greater number of sexual partners and failure to use condoms—place young people at heightened danger of contracting STIs (Kirby, 2007) and of passing on an STI to others in the sexual network of partners. There is new and important research on how sexually transmitted diseases spread. Kirby summarized the contours of risk:

> At the individual level, *the relationship between number of partners and probability of transmission is roughly linear. That is, having four sexual partners poses roughly twice the risk of contracting an STD as having two partners, other things being equal. Conversely, having two sexual partners instead of four reduces the risk by roughly half.* At the population level, *however, the potential for transmission increases exponentially. That is, small increases in the number of partners can greatly increase the risk of STD because they greatly increase the number of people who are connected to each other in sexual networks; conversely, small decreases in the number of partners can greatly decrease the risk. (p. 40)*

In the face of alarming rates of incidence of STIs among adolescents, especially girls, it is increasingly important to include the reduction of numbers of concurrent and total sexual partners among intervention objectives.

Overall, it is clear that the quality of the interaction of partners significantly affects the whole course of an individual's sexual life. In relationships of longer duration, where young women experience equality of power, young men support use of contraception, and they have discussed birth control, partners are more likely to use contraception (Kirby, 2001). Couples in such relationships are less likely to use condoms, but more likely to use another method to avoid unplanned pregnancy. Steadier relationships in which the couple communicates better are more characteristic of older adolescents. The capacity to be engaged in this kind of relationship increases with emotional and cognitive development, one of the reasons why younger teenagers are at greater risk of becoming pregnant if they are sexually active, and why it is best for young people to delay sexual initiation until they are fully capable of making positive choices that will support their health.

Community Environment

Community Disadvantage and Disorganization The highest rates of teenage pregnancy and childbearing occur among young people living in communities that are most economically disadvantaged, socially disorganized, and physically deteriorated. In the aggregate, residents in these communities have disproportionately high levels of unemployment, school dropout, divorce, single-parent families, teenage pregnancy and childbearing, crime, and residential turnover. They have lower levels of educational attainment, income, and religious involvement. In such communities, young people are more likely to have sexual intercourse earlier and without birth control and to become pregnant (Hogan & Kitagawa, 1985; Brewster, Billy, & Grady, 1993; Billy, Brewster, & Grady, 1994; Ku, Sonenstein, & Pleck, 1994; Lauritsen, 1994; Upchurch, Aneshense, Sucoff, & Levy-Storms, 1998; Kirby, 2007).

Although rates of teen pregnancy declined recently among minority youths living in poor neighborhoods, they have risen recently and remain, as a group, at the highest risk of early childbearing. According to some estimates, more than 70% of black children in some poor neighborhoods are born to unmarried women, including 30% to adolescents (Moore & Chase-Lansdale, 1999). There is a large multidisciplinary literature that examines why rates of early childbearing outside of marriage have risen so precipitously primarily among black young residents of poor, urban, and racially segregated neighborhoods.

However, because of historic racial residential segregation, "Hidden beneath the racial and geographic differences in all statistics in the United States lies the more serious and consistent association between adolescent conception and socioeconomic deprivation. . .the distribution pattern of adolescent births is essentially the same as those for infant mortality, homicide, and violent deaths among youth, violent crime and illicit drug use, all problems of high prevalence in poor and socially disadvantaged areas" (Hardy & Zabin, 1993, p. 52).

The precise ways in which community and neighborhood residence are related to young people's sexual behavior and fertility outcomes is extremely complex, and researchers now are only beginning to empirically disentangle their interconnections. There is increasing evidence that family structure and processes and extrafamilial social relationships interact within the neighborhood context to influence whether and how early young women and men begin to have sex (Moore & Chase-Lansdale, 1999; Upchurch et al., 1999). It is clear that, as Upchurch et al. (1999) observed, ". . .the risk of becoming sexually active is not solely due to the SES and race/ethnicity composition of the neighborhood but rather it is the social conditions that covary with these structural attributes that are important" (p. 930). In addition to family characteristics, some research finds that young people's perceptions of the safety, physical deterioration, and degree of social organization all have some impact on youths' sexual behavior (Kirby, 2007).

Although we tend to associate the typical social conditions associated within impoverished communities with urban settings, poor rural communities, such as the one in which Terry grew up in North Carolina, often share these features and also have high rates of pregnancy and parenthood among teens of all racial and ethnic backgrounds (South Carolina Campaign, 2000). Although we know that rural poverty is associated with teen pregnancy, few studies have examined whether and how the rural context is distinctive in its mechanisms of influence on young people's sexual and reproductive behavior.

Summary

The factors reviewed here are located at various distances from the individual adolescent's internal world. Individual factors or antecedents are closest, or most proximal, to sexual behaviors. They include the teen's own attitudes, values, and actions, and biological features that impinge on his or her sexuality-related choices. As we move away from the individual's own characteristics to the family and sociocultural environment, the risk factors or antecedents are more distal, or nonsexual. These have more indirect, but not necessarily weaker, impact on adolescents' sexual behavior. To target teen pregnancy prevention efforts to have greatest impact, it is important to know (a) how antecedent factors influence sexual behavior, and (b) to identify correctly what factors are present in adolescents' lives. In the following chapter, we will examine how antecedent risk factors contribute to levels of risky behavior in a continuum of risk.

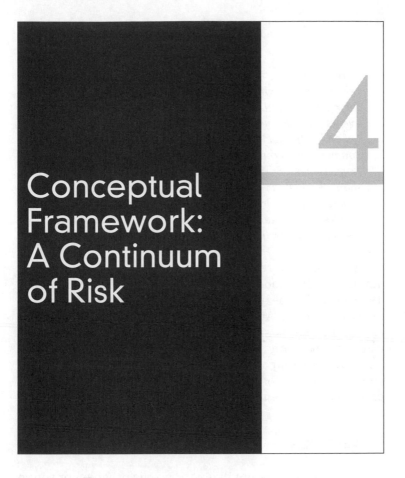

Conceptual Framework: A Continuum of Risk

Chapter 3 identified specific factors most strongly associated with young people engaging in risky sexual behaviors leading to early pregnancy and childbearing. How do these factors influence adolescents' sexual decisions? The integration of these factors does not lead to a single theory providing a comprehensive explanation for all teenagers. Rather, together the findings suggest that young women and men can be located on a continuum of risk according to their individual life experiences, characteristics, and social context.

In her synthesis of research on overall psychosocial risks among adolescents, Dryfoos visualizes "the life histories of the various risk groups in this way":

A train is leaving the station. Some children are born on the train and stay on until they grow up. They have supportive parents and live in a healthy community with a good school. Some children who are born on the train fall off of it because their families fall apart, or the school fails, or other stressful events occur. Some children are not born on the train and never get on it. They lack parental support, live in a poor social environment, drop out of terrible schools, and are surrounded by hopelessness. Some children are not born on the train but they manage to climb on it. These are the children that Rutter and others call "invulnerable" and "resilient." Almost always these children have had access to a caring individual who assisted them (not necessarily a parent). (Dryfoos, 1990, p. 109)

The ability to remain on this train toward "responsible adulthood" (Dryfoos, 1990, p. 109; Masten, Hubbard, Gest, Tellegen, & Garmezy, 1999) is well within the expectations of many, if not most, American youth. Nevertheless, derailment caused by events such as early pregnancy or parenthood threatens too many young people. For some, the threat looms large and encompassing, while for other more fortunate youths it consists of manageable and expectable challenges of normal development in contemporary society.

Lowest Risk

Most adolescents are not likely to become pregnant or young parents because they do not possess multiple serious environmental risk factors associated with early sex and other high-risk behaviors. At the same time, the average teenager today is exposed to cultural forces that encourage young people to behave in adult ways that leave them vulnerable to unwanted consequences such as pregnancy and, of increasing concern, sexually-transmitted diseases. Perhaps the most pervasive sources of risk among most teens result from a mismatch in the contemporary cultural expectations for mature decision making in a range of important arenas, such as sexuality, in relation to adolescents' capacities to meet those expectations. Consequently, the most significant antecedents among low-risk youths can be categorized mainly as *sexual or proximal*—that is, directly related to their attitudes and beliefs about sex and contraception, and their ability to form and act effectively on health-enhancing behavioral intentions.

Age significantly influences adolescents' capacities to meet these expectations.

In general, the younger the teen engages in sexual intercourse, the greater the chance of having an unintended pregnancy. One major reason (among those teens whose sexual activity is voluntary) is that he or she is less likely to predict accurately the consequences of his or her behavior. Development from early to middle adolescence is accompanied by a transition to formal operations that involve cognitive egocentrism, which results in a "personal fable" (Farber, 1994; Lapsley, 1993). Lapsley (1993) summarizes the elements of the concept:

> *According to this view, a young adolescent fails to differentiate what is the object of his or her own concern (e.g., the self) from the concerns and preoccupations of others, assuming, egocentrically, that others share one's own preoccupation with the self. One consequence of cognitive egocentrism is the tendency to construct* personal fables, *which are modes of self-understanding that include themes of* invulnerability *(the self is incapable of being harmed or injured),* omnipotence *(viewing the self as a source of special authority or influence), or* personal uniqueness *(the perspective of the self is so special it cannot be understood, "No one understands me!"). (p. 26)*

Elkind (Elkind and Bowen, 1979) and others traditionally view the personal fable as a primary source of miscalculation of potential personal consequences underlying risky sexual behavior among younger teens. Because of developmentally normal cognitive processes, when faced with the decision of whether to have unprotected intercourse, they may underestimate their own chances of "getting caught." Most young teens can understand—and state with accuracy—that having sexual intercourse without using birth control may result in someone becoming pregnant.

Lapsley (2003) challenges the assumption of the personal fable as a singular construct whose significance is solely a source of vulnerability to harm. He argues that the personal fable should be understood as one among a "family of 'positive illusions'" that can increase adaptive functioning in the face of the many psychological, emotional, and social demands of adolescent development (p. 27). He suggests that each type of fable can function either as protection against negative outcomes; for example, depression, or enhancer of health-compromising behavior, such as smoking or unprotected sex. This critique provides a more nuanced, and thus realistic, understanding of the complex processes of adolescent development and suggests the need for more differential assessment of individuals' functioning in a developmental context. At the same time, the common pattern of reasoning, in which younger teenagers minimize their personal risks, is that they are less likely than older adolescents to use contraception effectively. It is also one reason why only providing information about sexual risk-taking is not a very effective means of influencing the behavior of most young people.

Steinberg (2003) highlights additional reasons for caution in assuming that teens' risky choices are primarily the result of inadequate information. He suggests that "decision making" is too cognitively limited a concept to capture the reality of how adolescents evaluate relative risk. Rather, it is more accurate to consider the role of judgment in behavior, and teens are, in essence, more immature than adults in their judgment of what is appropriate. According to this perspective, even in possession of similar knowledge about the consequences, teens are more influenced by peer pressure, more oriented to the present than future, and less able to inhibit their impulses than are adults.

Adolescents, then, tend to have common developmental characteristics that affect how they process information and make behavioral choices. However, if the basic contours of development have not changed significantly over time, the same cannot be said for the swirling external forces of the environment in which these choices are made. Many behaviors, such as sexual intercourse, that were once considered appropriate only for adults have been defined "downward" chronologically; adolescence as a stage of social development has also been extended, with the age of marriage rising and more youths remaining in school longer. Despite significant changes in the social context of individual development, the common and predictable processes that characterize adolescence and the ways in which these biological, psychological, and social processes unfold in our current social context leave teens more vulnerable to early and unplanned pregnancy than in the past. In addition, these developmental processes influence teens' parenting practices. As this social reality has changed, so has our understanding of the nature of adolescence as a stage of development.

Following the seminal work of G. Stanley Hall in 1904, developmental theory characterized adolescence as a time of crisis. Blos (1962) explained the nature of the adolescent crisis as:

> . . . the sum total of all attempts at adjustment to the stage of puberty, to the new set of inner and outer—endogenous and exogenous—conditions which confront the individual. The urgent necessity to cope with the novel condition of puberty evokes all the modes of excitation, tension, gratification, and defense that ever played a role in previous years—that is during the psychosexual development of infancy and early childhood. This infantile admixture is responsible for the bizarreness and the regressive character of adolescent behavior; it is the typical expression of the adolescent struggle to regain or to retain a psychic equilibrium which has been jolted by the crisis of puberty. (p. 11)

The assumption of "adolescent immaturity" (Elkind, 1994, p. 148) was elaborated by Erikson in terms of the developmental tasks that required resolution for normal movement into adulthood. Primary among these tasks is the attainment of personal identity, the failure of which may result in role diffusion. Erikson believed that developing stable identity required a "moratorium, a kind of sabbatical from grown-up responsibilities and pressures to make important decisions about their lives" (Elkind, 1994, p. 149).

This view of the developmental needs of adolescents was consonant with what Elkind (1994) termed the "modern" family of the first 6 decades of the 20th century, in which parents expressed clear expectations for their children's values and behavior and provided strong guidance. He contrasted modern culture with the current "postmodern" society that has emerged since the 1960s. In today's "permeable" families, adults exert less authority over their children, leaving teenagers far more on their own to navigate the growing psychological, sexual, and occupational demands of our complex society:

> Now that we have moved into the postmodern era, the modern saga of adolescent immaturity is out of date. . .In its stead, a new perception has been created: teenage sophistication. We

now look upon adolescents as worldly-wise in matters of sex, drugs, music, computers, and consumerism. The teen years are no longer seen as a period of training for adult life; they are considered to be, rather a different form of adult life, with its own unique indices of maturity. (p. 148)

In this postmodern culture, children must begin their identity formation before their teenage years to cope with the vastly increased exposure to information and stimuli from the world outside of the family. We have hardly begun to understand the impact of pervasive forms of media, such as the internet on youth development.

Although adolescents may, in fact, be more capable of mature decision making than was suggested in earlier developmental theory, Elkind is correct in his observation that adolescents need more direction from adults than many receive today. Despite the fact that contemporary teenagers are increasingly knowledgeable about sexual matters and are encouraged by popular culture to see themselves as explicitly sexual beings, they are not yet adults because:

. . .in many respects, the adolescent transition is unique. Unlike adulthood, it is a period of extremely rapid physical, emotional, psychological, and social growth. This period of rapid growth leads to a metamorphosis unlike any transition that occurs in adulthood. Adult transitions take place within a relatively fixed firmament of physique, mental ability, and established social roles. Adolescent transitions do not. Even though young people are now exposed to demands for identity formation from an early age, they still need time in adolescence to adjust to their new body configuration, their new emotions, their new thinking abilities, and their new patterns of social interaction. (Elkind, 1994, p. 152)

Florence Lieberman (1973) observed that these essential developmental characteristics placed adolescent girls at particular risk in the context of the sexual "liberation" of the 1960s and 1970s. She described young women's dilemma in an increasingly sexualized society in which parents' own ambivalence prevents them from providing secure guidance:

Today virginity is devalued. So much so, as sexual activity is possible without conception, that much of society acts as if no female past the age of twelve is or should be virginal. The virgin adolescent, herself, is torn in three directions: the pressures of her peers, male and female, to dispense with the useless hymen; to be good and to please her parents, at any rate some of them, by remaining virginal until marriage; or to obey her inner feelings and to wait to develop the social, intellectual, and psychological strengths that will enable her to engage in sexual activities with security and pleasure. Only the last is a liberated choice. (p. 227)

The formative nature of adolescents' identity and all cognitive, emotional, and physical correlates of developing maturity create challenges for many teens in dealing constructively with the pressures for adult activities that exist all around them. The challenge of meeting these demands is exacerbated by the relatively great individual freedom expected by adults and youths in our society. In addition to the "high degree of plasticity" (Blos, 1962 p. 9) typical of adolescence, American society does not provide youth well-structured rites of passage to learn and practice how to respond to strong external pressures. In the context of little formal cultural patterning, the individual adolescent is left to "achieve by personal resourcefulness the adaptation that institutionalization does not offer him" (Blos, 1962, p. 9). When these intense pressures combine with weak direction from parents and other close adults, teenagers are left, in Elkind's words, to find their own way to adulthood.

Among the many demands for independent adaptation is the almost ubiquitous presence of various forms of media that portray sexual behavior openly and often glorify nonmarital sex. Distinct from the moral aspect of sex outside of marriage is the problem that the sexual images bombarding adolescents do not adequately distinguish between what is and what is not age-appropriate behavior for teenagers. Many teenagers thus assume that sexual intercourse is appropriate for people of any age and regardless of marital status. Nonmarital sex has simply become regarded by many youths—and adults—as a normal adolescent activity that serves to satisfy the common need for acceptance by peers and experimentation with adult roles.

Despite the strong positive messages teens receive from peers and the public media about sexual activity, many teens feel deeply ambivalent about having sex. In addition to experiencing moral conflict, many teenagers simply feel emotionally or physically unprepared or even scared of having sex.

Young women and men who have sex often do not enjoy and even regret their decision even if they do not suffer adverse physical consequences, such as conceiving or contracting an STI (Elkind, 1994; Farber, 1992). As one middle-class white teen mother reflected so poignantly:

> . . .when I had sex, when I was like 14 with that guy, I didn't enjoy it. I didn't know what I was doing, and that gets me pissed that some of these [other] girls are gonna have to go through what I went through. . . It's worth it if you can handle it, but some girls just can't handle it. You don't have to do it. . .it's not worth all the pain and suffering that you go through if you do get pregnant. It's not worth hurting a child if you do keep it. . .it's not worth thinking about what your future could have been; thinking about how it would be if it was with a guy you were really in love with. There's just too many things. . . (Farber, 1992, p. 72)

Young people's mixed feelings—of wanting to fit in, to be accepted and liked but not being ready for the actual experience or feeling guilty—can decrease their effective use of birth control (Becker, 1998, p. 40). So that, although the cognitive capacity to prevent pregnancy in a planned way increases over the course of adolescence, even older teens ostensibly not at high risk of pregnancy may face barriers to prevention if they become sexually active. Many of the most frequently named reasons for having unprotected intercourse, such as not planning to have sex or allowing it to "just happen," reflect some teens' reluctance to take conscious responsibility for their sexual activity. Whether the source of their ambivalence lies in values of the family, community or religion, or in individual emotional development, the fact remains that they are taking profoundly serious actions often without feeling equipped to handle the potential consequences.

In general, low-risk youths possess sufficient motivation to make decisions that will ensure their educational and occupational success, including avoiding young parenthood. Such motivation is strengthened by receiving support for positive choices from adults at home and in their communities. However, they require knowledge about human sexuality, including the consequences of risky behavior, such as STIs, AIDS, and pregnancy, to make informed decisions about sexual relationships and contraception that are consistent with their most important values and life goals. In the sexualized environment in which most American adolescents live, many lack the decision-making and social skills necessary to act on the more health-producing decisions of which they are capable. Providing such knowledge and skills should be the prevention objectives for services to low-risk young men and women.

Moderate To High Risk

Beyond the generalized pressures to behave as sexually mature adults, some young people face greater vulnerability to early pregnancy and childbearing because individual family and personal characteristics lead them to engage in various high-risk behaviors including—but not limited to—unprotected sexual intercourse. Like most other American youths, they grow up in a sexualized society that demands greater emotional and cognitive maturity than many young people possess. However, unlike teens at low risk, these young people generally do not have strong environmental support to nurture positive and healthful personal decisions. Their risk of early, unprotected sexual activity often is part of those conditions that motivate them to participate in delinquent acts, use drugs and alcohol, and/or do poorly in school (Huizinga, Loeber, & Thornberry, 1993). Engaging in high-risk sexual activity thus has different meaning for these youths than it does for those at lower risk of pregnancy.

Among the sexual and nonsexual conditions that lead young people to risk their health and their futures, six antecedent characteristics place young people at especially significant risk of engaging in several related problem behaviors (Dryfoos, 1991, p. 109). These characteristics include (a) early age of initiation of the behaviors, (b) low expectations for and poor performance in school, (c) engagement in general problem behaviors, such as various forms of acting out, antisocial behavior, and other conduct disorders, (d) being easily influenced by peers who participate in problem behaviors, (e) weak parental bonding, and (f) residence in poor or dense urban neighborhood.

Many emotionally troubled young women and men engage in early and unprotected sexual intercourse along with other problem behaviors that threaten their well-being.

Dryfoos describes ways in which these problem behaviors are interrelated:

1. Delinquency is associated with early sexual activity, early pregnancy, substance abuse, low grades, and dropping out.
2. Early initiation of smoking and alcohol leads to heavier use of cigarettes and alcohol, and also leads to the use of marijuana and other illicit drugs.
3. Heavy substance abuse is associated with early sexual activity, lower grades, dropping out, and delinquency.
4. Early initiation of sexual activity is related to the use of cigarettes and alcohol, use of marijuana and other illicit drugs, lower grades, dropping out, and delinquency.
5. Early childbearing is related to early sexual activity, heavy drug use, low academic achievement, dropping out, and delinquency.
6. School failure leads to dropping out. Lower grades are associated with substance abuse, dropping out, and delinquency.
7. The number of risky behaviors that are engaged in is strongly related to the seriousness of the problems that result from the behaviors (Dryfoos, 1990).

Ensminger (1987) identified three major theoretical perspectives about why some youths are more likely than others to participate in these high-risk or problem behaviors. First, in their groundbreaking research, Jessor and Jessor (1977) identified sexual activity as one of several deviant behaviors constituting a "syndrome" of problem behaviors, also including use of marijuana and alcohol and general expressions of nonconformism. The *problem behavior theory* of Jessor and others views early sex, substance abuse, and delinquency as developmentally off-course efforts to make the transition to adulthood. Proneness to problem behavior is evident in the adolescent's personality, perceived environment, and actual behavior. Factors that increase such proneness include high value on independence and low expectations for academic goals, low support and control from significant others and approval and models for engaging in problem behavior, and low involvement in conventional behaviors, such as church attendance and school performance.

A second perspective that views teens' sexual activity as an aspect of overall deviance is *social control theory*. Hirschi (1969) identified four aspects of social bonds that inhibit deviant behavior: attachment to others, commitment (dedication to pursuing conventional objectives), involvement in structural activities, and conventional beliefs. According to this view, adolescents who are less attached to societal institutions, such as family, school, or peer group are more likely to deviate from conventional norms. Regardless of those to whom a child is attached, it is that attachment itself that protects a youth from acting unconventionally.

A third framework views differently the influence of significant members of individuals' social environments. According to *socialization* or *social learning theories*, adolescents are highly influenced by the modeling effect of those in their families, peer groups, and school contexts. Thus, if a teenager lives with a parent who uses drugs, or has sexual relations outside of marriage, he or she is likely to follow suit. Conversely, closely associating and identifying with others who do not engage in high-risk behavior supports young people who make healthy and prosocial choices about their own behavior.

The latter two perspectives are based on *social learning theory*, currently a highly popular theoretical basis for pregnancy and HIV/STI prevention programs of various types. Its tenets inform a range of program activities designed to provide youths a positive peer group experience that explicitly supports sexual abstinence and low-risk sexual behavior. Creating "alternative" peer group norms is believed to be especially useful for young men and women in high-risk social environments in which risky sex is normative and positively sanctioned.

Ravoira and Cherry (1992) applied these theories in their attempt to understand the sexual motivations of pregnant and parenting runaway and homeless girls. They conclude that when young women have weak attachments to "society," they are more likely to behave in ways that dramatically depart from age-appropriate social norms. They conceive of these attachments in terms of the strength of girls' social bonds to important others, such as family, friends, and the community, and conclude that the stronger the bonds, the less deviant their behavior.

For young women and men who are either at significant risk of early sex and pregnancy because they are already engaging in other risky behavior, or possess multiple characteristics associated with general high-risk behavior, providing knowledge about how to prevent pregnancy is not adequate.

Insofar as adolescents' high-risk sexual activity expresses low commitment to conventional achievement, or emotional distress, or the presence of deviant social norms, they may have little motivation to avoid unprotected sex or even pregnancy. Whitaker, Miller, and Clark (2000) urge program planners to differentiate between youths who do not intend to have sex in the near future and those at higher risk who anticipate being sexually active. For the latter group, ". . . riskier sexual experiences occur in a unique social and psychological context, which may be evident even before teenagers begin to engage in sex. . .Interventions must better address factors such as peer norms, parenting and connections to institutions such as school and religion that may motivate adolescents to delay sexual activity" (Whitaker et al., 2000, p. 116).

Pregnancy prevention for these young people should address the multiple antecedents associated with a range of high-risk behaviors. Appropriate program objectives will include not only increasing teens' knowledge and skills, but also the intention to apply the knowledge and skills to reducing their risk-taking.

Highest Risk

Despite the decline in fertility among teens who have experienced the highest fertility rates, those at greatest risk of early unprotected sex and pregnancy continue to be youths growing up in poverty amid general community and family chaos. The nature of these antecedent conditions also places young people at risk of the most negative outcomes of teen pregnancy. The severity of this risk is not simply a sum of individual risk factors discussed above. These factors are generally present, but often in a particular social context that may positively sanction early childbearing (Burton, 1990).

For many very poor young people, avoiding early pregnancy and parenthood can be a form of social deviance. Consequently, prevention efforts for the highest-risk youths must address the full range of sexual and nonsexual antecedents throughout all environmental levels to be effective.

Contemporary sociocultural theories emphasize the overwhelming impact of economic and social structures on the motivation of poor teens to avoid early childbearing. Unlike youths whose high-risk behavior departs from the mainstream norms of their social environment, early sex, pregnancy, and childbearing are more culturally syntonic in deeply impoverished and distressed communities. Much recent research on the most disadvantaged youth draws from the seminal work of economist Gary Becker and colleagues in the 1970s on *Utility Maximization and the Marriage Market* (Becker & Michael, 1977). Based on the assumption that individuals act "rationally" in calculating the costs and benefits of their decisions—including marriage and childbearing—numerous researchers have hypothesized an overall decline in gains from marriage among young people in impoverished communities (Wilson, 1987; Hopkins, 1987). This economic perspective informs the popular "opportunity cost" analysis of teen pregnancy, suggesting that teens who allow themselves to become pregnant and choose motherhood perceive less "cost" to their futures than do teens who avoid pregnancy.

Why do these youths feel that they have so little to lose in future educational and occupational achievement by becoming single teen parents? One view attributes rising teenage illegitimacy to increased availability of public assistance that began during the 1960s. Charles Murray, whose once-controversial views have largely prevailed in the form of the 1996 welfare reform, argued that increasing illegitimacy among poor youth was directly attributable to perverse incentives of welfare programs like AFDC that rewarded nonmarital childbearing and discouraged marriage (Murray, 1984). There is little empirical evidence that particular welfare programs have a direct impact on marital choices, or on sexual and parenting behavior (Edin & Lein, 1997; Moffitt, 1992; Nathan, Gentry, & Lawrence, 1999). In addition, others point out that because the real value of benefits, such as AFDC, actually declined over time, the "generosity" of welfare could not have been an incentive for rising out-of-wedlock among teenagers (Danziger, 1994; Burtless, 1994).

Among the explicit objectives of the TANF legislation was the reduction of pregnancy and out-of-wedlock childbearing among teens. It is too early to know the actual impact of TANF on adolescent fertility, but Furstenberg (2007) argues that the problems associated with adolescent fertility and family formation increasingly are the problems of poverty. Thus, he concludes, "The fact is that while early childbearing has declined and welfare as we know it, has been eliminated, the problem of economic disadvantage has hardly changes at all" (p. 159).

Nevertheless, there has been little research that explores how generations of living in chronic poverty and relying on public assistance may have shaped individuals' expectations and habits over time so as to virtually separate marriage and childbearing among many poor young people.

Another influential macro perspective on the motivations of poor teenagers to have children outside of marriage emphasizes how recent changes in the structure of urban economies have diminished the opportunities for blue-collar employment that once allowed working-class men to support their families. In the influential *The Truly Disadvantaged*, William Julius Wilson (1987) hypothesized that the high proportion of black men who are incarcerated and die young from the violence that plagues impoverished inner-city communities combined with minimal legitimate economic opportunity to create a reduced "male marriageable pool" available to black women. Many young women in physically and culturally isolated communities perceive limited educational, occupational, and marital opportunities. With no realistic expectation of either upward mobility or marriage, they sacrifice little by having children as unmarried teenagers. In this situation, as Rainwater observed nearly 20 years before, having a child provides a source of love while providing a way of making the transition to adulthood.

These two perspectives are associated with quite divergent policy and micropractice implications if they are taken as sole explanatory models. In reality, they are not mutually exclusive. Certainly, there has been a decline in economic opportunity for individuals with low levels of education and skills that has also diminished the capacity of many men to provide adequately for their families. Ethnographic research has documented how the ability of many young men and women to form stable and lasting marital unions has eroded in economically deteriorated communities (Burton, 1990). Consequently, in the context of few other options, we now see two, three, and even more generations of unmarried women who have relied upon public assistance to support their children.

There are clear associations between lack of economic opportunity and early out-of-wedlock childbearing; yet, it is difficult to disentangle meaningfully the effects of community poverty, public policies, and cultural changes wrought over years of increasing social and economic decay when a teenager risks pregnancy by having unprotected sex.

One methodological challenge is identifying mechanisms by which larger cultural or structural features of a society affect individuals' behavior on a daily basis or in an intimate interpersonal context. Burton (1990) suggests how social forces have led to the perpetuation of intergenerational female-headed families and teenage childbearing as an "alternative strategy" to marriage and adult childbearing among low-income blacks. This strategy is characterized by an accelerated family timetable, the separation of reproduction and marriage, and a grandparental child-rearing system. Burton asserts that this alternative family formation is an adaptation to high rates of black male unemployment, the preferences of black men for white women, the assignment of "designated" teenage childbearers, grandmothers' needs to fulfill parenting desires, and a "skip-generation" pattern of family caregiving and dependency. Thus, in the tradition of cultural relativists, Burton views teenage and out-of-wedlock childbearing as a bona fide cultural pattern, adapting to and reinforced by social and economic structures and consciously passed down to succeeding generations of young women.

Though Burton's analysis provides a plausible set of explanatory factors for teen childbearing, it leaves unexplored many deeper issues of personal motivation. The difficulty in identifying what are the most important influences is more than simply one of research methods; it reflects how profoundly intertwined are the forces of the psyche with the many external realities that make up any individual's life space. Anne Dean (1997), in her study of adolescent motherhood in a poor, southern rural community concludes:

> *The most important message to be taken from this work is that what motivates people in this community with respect to the adolescent pregnancy behavior pattern is not the environments per se, but how people interpret and understand at varying levels of their conscious and unconscious minds what environments and actions mean for themselves as individuals and as members of a social or cultural group. Environments, one might say, are where some of the action is; the rest is with the individuals and groups of individuals who feel, experience, act in and interpret environment. (p. 188)*

Dean compared teenage mothers with other young women and found differences in their personal and cultural "schemas" that defined "hierarchies of goals and means of achieving them" (Dean, 1997, p. 192). These schemas, or systems of personal meaning, led the young women in divergent directions, either toward marriage, work, and away from their impoverished community, or inward to their own mothers with limited resources and to the lives that were familiar and required little personal change. These choices limit the future of the young mothers and their children:

> The point is not that children growing up in single-parent households cannot develop favorably. . . The point is, rather, that mothers in downwardly mobile environments lack the support of extended families, lack the emotional and economic support of a husband, lack sufficient and reliable resources for caring for themselves and for their children, and are likely themselves to have constructed deprived working models of their own attachment relationships . . . In this kind of social and psychological environment, the difficulties for the mother-child dyad of negotiating a path toward psychological maturity are greatly increased. The consequences of failing to do so include among others the increased likelihood of adolescent pregnancy for children who become adolescents, greater difficulty forming and maintaining a stable relationship with a partner, and greater difficulties taking advantage of increased opportunities for social and economic advancement. These outcomes then feed back into the system and the downward spiral continues. (Dean, 1997, p. 195)

A similar observation that so many disadvantaged young mothers and those at risk of teen pregnancy do not benefit from social programs led Judith Musick to assess patterns of development of poor inner city adolescent mothers. She acknowledges the "cumulative effects of poverty on the family," (Musick, 1993, p. 61), but seeks a deeper understanding of the relationship between the environmental stresses of poverty and intrapsychic processes of adaptation. Describing how the development of girls raised in severe poverty is compromised, Musick observes:

> These girls frequently have grown up in damaged and damaging family situations where the basic developmental foundation has been poorly laid or is lacking altogether. In addition, the environment in which they live—at home,

in school, and in the community—is often highly threaten-ing. Surely more of these teens, when compared with their more advantaged counterparts, are highly stressed if not deeply troubled. At the same time, their external supports and their opportunities to find alternative models of coping are few and far less adequate. (p. 59)

Mature development requires resolving common iden-tity-related issues through stages of adolescence. Many poor girls who do not experience consistent parental nurturing because of environmental deficiency, violence, and other threats to security remain fixed on issues more characteristic of early adolescence. Sexual acting out then often results in pregnancy and motherhood:

If an adolescent's psychological energies are too strongly focused on defensive and security measures, much of her time and effort will be focused on trying to resolve her unmet dependency needs, searching for and trying to main-tain attachments. When this occurs, her attention and ener-gies are diverted from the critical developmental tasks that undergird adolescent and, later, adult competence in our society. Girls for whom basic acceptance and love are the primary motivating forces have little interest or emotional energy to invest in school of work-related activities unless they are exceptionally bright or talented. Even then, the pull of unmet affiliative or dependency needs may be more pow-erful than anything the worlds of school or work have to offer, particularly when these offerings are as inadequate and inconsistent as those typically found in poverty com-munities. (Musick, 1993, p. 61)

To avoid teenage motherhood in this context of severe environmental deficiencies, a girl requires "not just average but above-average psychological resources and strengths, self-concepts, and competencies" (Musick, 1993, p. 13).

The psychological dynamics that contribute to poor teens' risk of early pregnancy also exacerbate the negative consequences that so often follow adolescent motherhood. If girls in more affluent families suffer from unmet emotional needs, their greater resources and environmental supports can mitigate the worst long-term results in their own and their children's development and well-being. In contrast, poorer girls are less likely to recover from the emotional distress and the educational and occupational losses that may accompany an early pregnancy.

Summary

The concept of differential risk based on a range of individual and contextual characteristics has direct implications for teen pregnancy prevention. Only by identifying closely the sources of risk can we target efforts most effectively and efficiently; only by so doing can we develop prevention programs that respond directly to the antecedent factors exerting the strongest influence on young people's sexual risk-taking.

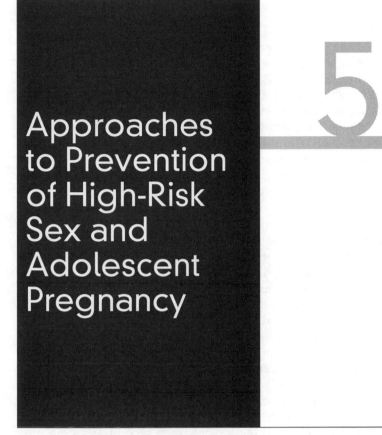

Approaches to Prevention of High-Risk Sex and Adolescent Pregnancy

5

Chapter 4 proposed a continuum of risk of teens engaging in early and unprotected sex, hence of pregnancy and of acquiring sexually transmitted infections (STIs). Teens who are most vulnerable to pregnancy and to STI experience the greatest number of risk factors and, conversely, the fewest protective factors. In addition, the risk factors exist at all levels of their sociocultural environments. In general, the more numerous the risks and the more broadly the risk factors extend outward from the individual to the community, the more severe the level of risk he or she faces. This information forms an essential base in designing prevention strategies that respond effectively to the particular antecedent conditions to early and risky sexual activity. The main focus of prevention here is early pregnancy, with secondary attention to preventing contracting STI. Effective prevention of STI by definition can reduce conception, most directly through abstinence and use of condoms, whereas the inverse is not necessarily true. That is because using other methods of birth control do not protect against STI. Thus, discussion of teen pregnancy prevention is best understood in its broadest meaning of reducing high-risk sexual activity. This expansive conceptualization increasingly informs prevention programs that include reduction of both pregnancy and STI as ultimate outcome objectives.

The goals of primary pregnancy prevention are to help childless young women avoid becoming pregnant and to help young men avoid impregnating young women. Secondary prevention is directed toward averting subsequent pregnancy among women and men who have already borne or fathered children. Though teen parents have particular needs as individuals and as parents, research about prevention of subsequent pregnancy tends to be subsumed under discussions of prevention among highest-risk youths. Because the conditions contributing to the greatest risk of a first pregnancy generally remain or are exacerbated after becoming a teen parent, secondary prevention here is both implicitly included in discussion of needs of high-risk young people and will be explicitly addressed in chapter 9. Primary prevention of STI refers to avoiding initial infection, whereas secondary prevention includes avoiding subsequent infection (after treatment) of the same or another STI.

Pregnancy can deliberately be avoided mainly one of two ways: by abstaining from sexual intercourse or by using birth control during sexual intercourse. Whether public policies and prevention programs should advocate one or the other or both of these means is the subject of intense controversy whose resolution lies far beyond the question of which works best to prevent teenagers from conceiving. The very choices deeply touch the heart of social and personal values and beliefs. While few concerned adults disagree that prevention of pregnancy and disease are the proper goals, active dissention about the means can seriously hinder communities from promoting healthy youth development, including helping young people from taking unnecessary risks with their current and future well-being.

The extent to which decisions about these choices often are value based is evident in the strong preference by federal funding agencies for an abstinence-only approach to prevention. Although this position expresses genuine commitments of many Americans to abstinence education as the most desirable strategy, it does not reflect public consensus, nor is it based on knowledge from the best evaluation research that has become available in the past few years.

To make sound professional decisions about various approaches to adolescent pregnancy prevention, it is necessary to balance the deeply held values and preferences of varied community constituencies and organizational stakeholders with research-based information about the impact of particular interventions on young women's and men's sexual behavior. Achieving this balance requires both a thorough knowledge of approaches to prevention and sensitivity to the particular community context for which policies are designed and where services are delivered.

Types of Prevention Programs

Many types of pregnancy prevention programs exist within diverse service settings (Bennett & Assefi, 2005). They differ in the target ages and gender of their clients, the missions of the host agencies, their practice approaches, and many other contextual variables. Though all of these programs seek ultimately to reduce rates of pregnancy and STIs among teens, they usually have proximate behavioral objectives, such as delaying the initiation of sexual activity, decreasing the frequency of intercourse or the number of sexual partners or increasing intention to abstain from sex or attitudinal objectives that influence behavior (Monahan, 2001). Common strategies to achieve these objectives include changing adolescents' values, increasing sexuality-related information and skills, expanding life skills and options, and providing birth control. These strategies employ varied practice methods such as using standardized curricula, intensive counseling, service learning, and creating public awareness campaigns, among others.

Clearly, some approaches are more effective with certain groups of teens than with others (Dworkin, Harding, & Schreiber, 1993). However, there is room—there is need—for variety in methods of prevention spanning all levels of the environment. Such variety is necessary to respond to the many sources of teens' risk of pregnancy and STIs at different times in their development and to the preferences, values, and characteristics of teens, their families, and communities. In other words, there is no single magic bullet that will help all young people delay pregnancy and parenthood and avoid STI. Instead, there are many approaches that together can help reduce teens' high-risk sexual activity within a community. Increasingly, prevention is being understood as the responsibility of communities and not only single programs. That is, an "all fronts" effort is necessary to make meaningful change among young people's sexual behavior. However, this front is composed of individual programs in different settings whose success depends on targeting youths according to the degree and kinds of risks they face.

The wide array of prevention programs can be divided conceptually into three main categories: those that address primarily *sexual antecedents* directly, those that focus on *nonsexual antecedents*, and those that include *both sexual and nonsexual antecedents*. Programs within these broad categories may have quite different program objectives, philosophies, and practice approaches, or combine elements of each within a single program.

Discussions of prevention sometimes distinguish programs exclusively for young men. Although young men and women face some different gender-specific social pressures and developmental exigencies, many of their motivations for early and unprotected sex are similar. The following review assumes that program elements can—and should—be designed with sensitivity to gender where differences are indicated, but not necessarily built on fundamental theoretical differences regarding the mechanisms of behavior change. Similarly, while social workers increasingly attempt to incorporate principles of cultural diversity into practice, there is, unfortunately, relatively little in the current prevention literature that addresses cultural issues in any systematic way. This remains an important gap in our practice literature.

Sexual Antecedents

One main category of programs focuses mainly on sexual antecedents, those influences closest or most *proximal* to the individual's sexual behavior. Based broadly on cognitive behavioral and social learning principles of behavior change, they intervene in the processes that are directly under individual teenagers' control and directly affect their actual sexual behavior. Many programs focused on sexual antecedents either explicitly or implicitly draw on a core of theories such as theory of reasoned action, theory of planned behavior, transtheoretical model, developmental assets, and related theories discussed in chapter 3. They incorporate an individual-level perspective by focusing on teens' (a) attitudes toward and knowledge and beliefs about sex, birth control, and nonmarital childbearing; (b) their behavioral intentions; (c) their confidence in being able to act on those stated preferences; and (d) their actual skills in achieving desired ends.

There are several reasons to focus on these and other relevant attitudes and perceptions in prevention programs. First, the influence of all of these attitudes and perceptions together is direct and strong. Second, attitudes and perceptions are more immediately amenable to change than actual behavior. Third, they can also be identified and "measured" more easily than many other factors, especially those that are more environmentally distant from the individual. Consequently, sexual psychosocial antecedents to sexual behavior are frequently the explicit targets for change in pregnancy and HIV/STI prevention programs.

Programs addressing sexual psychosocial antecedents usually include some combination of the following specific objectives: (a) increasing youths' knowledge of human sexuality, including reproduction and birth control, (b) encouraging positive attitudes toward avoiding sex and/or protected sex, (c) enhancing behavioral skills such as refusing pressure to have sex or unprotected sex, (d) providing access to contraception, and (e) delaying the initiation of sexual activity and reducing the number of sexual partners. While these programs often share underlying theoretical assumptions about what leads to change in teens' sexual behavior, there are also major differences in the their orientations.

One important distinction is between programs that are exclusively "abstinence only" in contrast to programs that may teach abstinence but also provide knowledge and skills for teenagers who may become or are already sexually active, so-called *abstinence-plus* or comprehensive programs. Most programs fall somewhere in between the absolute position of teaching abstinence as the only permissible choice and an educational, value-free approach to human sexuality. Also, in response to requirements of many funding sources, community norms and other forces, many larger agencies—for example, those that serve both teen parents and those teens who have not been sexually active such as Rosalie Manor in Milwaukee (see http://www.rosaliemanor.org)—may include multiple approaches in the form of separate programs.

Abstinence-Only Education Abstinence-only education programs have received a great deal of public support as well as increasing scrutiny in recent years. They teach teenagers that abstaining from sex is the most effective and also the right way to prevent pregnancy and STIs (Masters, Beadnell, & Hoppe, 2008; Sather, & Zinn, 2002). These programs operate in many different venues such as schools, community agencies, health-related agencies, and religious organizations. Some programs focus solely on teaching the value of delaying sex until marriage, while other programs also include information about contraception but emphasize the potential for contraceptive failure and do not teach skills for using birth control. (Goodson, Pruitt, Suther, Wilson, & Buhi, 2006; Wilson, Goodson, Pruitt. Buhi, & Davis-Gunnels, 2005). The emphasis in abstinence education is on primary prevention, though some programs use the notion of "secondary virginity" and include teens who were sexually active but may choose not to have sex again until they are married.

For several years, the federal government has endorsed abstinence education for teenagers as part of its initiative to decrease the overall incidence out-of wedlock childbearing. Section 510 of the Personal Responsibility and Work Opportunity Reconciliation Act of 1996 defined abstinence education, specified in the so-called "A-H guidelines" as that which:

A. Has as its excusive purpose, teaching the social, psychological and health gains to be realized by abstaining from sexual activity;
B. Teaches abstinence from sexual activity outside marriage as the expected standard for all school age children;
C. Teaches that abstinence from sexual activity is the only certain way to avoid out-of-wedlock pregnancy, sexually transmitted diseases, and other associated health problems;

D. Teaches that a mutually faithfully monogamous relationship in the context of marriage is the expected standard of human sexual activity;

E. Teaches that sexual activity outside of marriage is likely to have harmful psychological and physical effects;

F. Teaches that bearing children out-of-wedlock is likely to have harmful consequences for the child, the child's parents, and society;

G. Teaches young people how to reject sexual advances and how alcohol and drug use increases vulnerability to sexual advances; and

H. Teaches the importance of attaining self-sufficiency before engaging in sexual activity (Title V, Section 510 [b][2] [A-H] of the Social Security Act [P.L.104–193]).

Programs receiving funds under this legislation must adhere to these eight mandates to receive support from most federal funding sources.

Within the parameters of these guidelines, abstinence-until-marriage-only programs use various intervention methods that address sexual antecedents to young people becoming sexually active. Many use standardized curricula, such as *Sex Can Wait*, *Postponing Sexual Involvement*, or *Sex Respect*. These curricula characteristically include both didactic education and experiential techniques designed to encourage positive attitudes toward abstinence, increase intention to abstain from nonmarital sex, and develop the capacity to act on the intention not to have sex until marriage. Numerous curricula also address nonsexual antecedents such as self-esteem and general decision making.

Common topics in abstinence-only programs include physical development and reproduction, risk awareness, goal setting and decision making, and interpersonal and relationship skills (Maynard, R., Trenholm, C., Devaney, B., Johnson, A., Clark, M., Homrighausen, J., 2005, p. 8). A typical example of this combined focus is the *Sexual Safety Awareness Curriculum* (SSAC), described in an evaluation study as, ". . .ten 45-minute didactic and experiential sessions. The core curriculum elements focused on victimization theory, examination of power in relationships, and examination of control of students' feelings. The goals of SSAC were to help students maintain a stronger affiliation with values about sexual abstinence and to better understand the potential personal, health, and social consequences of sexual involve-ment" (Zanis, 2005, p. 60). Some programs also emphasize broader character education to support values that encour-age sexual abstinence. Other programs do not adopt the fed-eral guidelines and promote abstinence, but not necessarily until marriage; and still other abstinence programs include open and objective consideration of various types of birth control but discourage adopting the value of "safe sex" out-side of marriage.

Despite programmatic variation, abstinence programs tend to share some core assumptions (Barnett & Hurst, 2003; Doniger, Adams, Utter, & Riley, 2001). By defini-tion, those programs that receive funding from the major streams adhere to the tenets articulated in the A-H stan-dards. In addition to the value positions contained in the standards, most programs also assume theoretically a fundamental incompatibility between encouraging young people to abstain from sex until marriage and encourag-ing healthy and responsible sexual activity. Many advocates of abstinence-only education fear that providing the latter implicitly communicates a mixed message that condones adolescent sexual activity.

Some of the controversy surrounding abstinence educa-tion arises from the lack of scientific evidence regarding effec-tiveness and questions about potential bias in the content and presentation of ostensibly objective information used to support abstinence as a goal. Reflecting these concerns, the Government Accounting Office (GAO) was asked by Congress to assess the accuracy and effectiveness of abstinence edu-cation programs supported by the Department of Health and Human Services (HHS). The GAO conducted a wide-ranging review of efforts by HHS and states receiving abstinence education funding from HHS to assess their programs, in consultation with independent researchers. The 2006 report concluded that it was difficult to ascertain the effectiveness of abstinence-until-marriage education programs because most attempts "have not met certain minimum scientific criteria—such as random assignment of participants and sufficient follow up periods and sample sizes—that experts have concluded are necessary in order for assessment of program effectiveness to be scientifically valid. . ." (GAO, 2006, p. i). The report also found that there is weak oversight by key government granting agencies of scientific accuracy in the content of abstinence program materials, resulting in the inclusion of some incorrect statements about human physiology and reproduction (GAO, 2006, p. 5).

The results of methodologically sound evaluations of abstinence-only programs have been eagerly awaited and some information is now available. A sample of programs funded under Title V was rigorously evaluated by Mathematica Policy Research. Using an experimental design, the Mathematica evaluation included 2,057 youth who were randomly assigned to either a program or control group in one of four programs located in Powhatan, Virginia; Miami, Florida; Milwaukee, Wisconsin; or Clarksdale, Mississippi. The programs varied by their methods of service delivery (including setting, program type, and whether they had voluntary attendance), the ages of the participating youths, service duration and intensity, and availability of other services to youth. The outcomes included measures of behavior as well as knowledge and perceptions. The study found that program participants "were no more likely than control group youth to have abstained from sex, and, among those who reported having had sex, they had similar numbers of sexual partners and had initiated sex at the same mean age" (Devaney, Johnson, Maynard, and Trenholm, 2007, xvii). The programs did improve youths' knowledge of the risks of pregnancy and their ability to identify sexually transmitted diseases, "but had no overall impact on knowledge of unprotected sex risks and the consequences of STDs" (Devaney, et al., 2007, xviii). While there was significant disagreement about the legitimacy of these findings among various advocates for abstinence education, the study provides an important set of findings based on strong scientific methods.

In addition to this important evaluation study, several states have been conducting evaluations of their abstinence education programs (LeCroy, 2003). Taken together, there is now a substantial enough scientifically valid evaluation literature available to provide some guidance for using abstinence-only as a prevention approach. The weight of the most scientifically rigorous research suggests that abstinence-only programs do not have significant impact on the sexual behavior of participants over time (Borakowski, Trapl, Lovegreen, Colabianchi, & Block, 2005; Carter-Jessop, Fanklin, Heath, Jiminez-Irazarry, & Peace, 2000). Kirby (2007) summarizes the existing research on the effect of those abstinence programs using standardized curricula whose evaluations meet stringent criteria for methodological soundness plus a few less rigorously designed studies:

> *Several abstinence-until-marriage programs have been* rigorously *evaluated in experimental studies with large samples and found to have no overall impact on delay of initiation of sex, age of initiation, return to abstinence, number of sexual partners, or use of condoms or other contraceptives. (p. 102)*

Although there is not compelling evidence that counters this general conclusion, some caveats must be noted. First, findings from a few evaluations with more positive results have been presented at professional conferences but not yet published. Second, many programs have not been rigorously evaluated, so one cannot logically conclude that they do not have positive impact. Third, this nascent evidence-based literature includes many studies whose samples are not comparable in age and other methodological limitations associated with the wide range of programs defined as abstinence-only. Thus, one must be cautious about generalizing findings about abstinence-only programs to all adolescents.

It appears that there may be differential impact of abstinence-only education on young people that is also context specific. The "virginity pledge" taken by teenagers in some high schools, for example, does have at least some short-term influence on pledges' intentions to remain abstinent, but only when they remain in the minority among other students. The impact disappears when over a third of the student body makes the pledge. Another example of the challenge in drawing generalized valid conclusions is evident in research examining the impact of abstinence education on boys and girls of different ages and over time. One evaluation of the commonly used curriculum, *Sex Can Wait*, implemented with all age-group components, found weak but positive short- and long-term impact on knowledge, hopefulness, and self-efficacy among upper-elementary school students; no short-term but positive long-term behavioral impact among middle school students; and positive short-term behavioral impact that did not extend to the 18-month follow up (Denny & Young, 2006).

In summary, current knowledge suggests that abstinence-only programs can be slightly effective with boys and girls who are still virgins by increasing their knowledge about risks of early sexual activity and intention to remain abstinent longer than their peers. The older adolescents are, however, the less effective abstinence-only education is in affecting their actual sexual behavior. Abstinence-only programs may increase their knowledge about and attitudes toward sexuality and sexual behavior, but currently there is no evidence to suggest that alone they alter teens' actual sexual behavior so as to reduce their risk of conceiving or contracting STI (Trenholm, Devaney, Fortson, Clark, Quay, and Wheeler, 2008).

Another other major group of prevention programs that directly addresses sexual antecedents is comprehensive *sexuality and HIV/STD education programs*, also located in middle schools, high schools, and various types of community-based agencies (Bennett & Asseif, 2005). These programs typically teach that abstinence is the best choice for preventing pregnancy and sexually transmitted infections (STIs) but also provide education about alternatives for having "safe sex." Most of the abstinence-plus programs also use standardized curricula such as *Making Proud Choices! A Safer Sex Curriculum; Safer Choices, Becoming a Responsible Teen,* or *Making a Difference: A Safer Sex Approach to STD, Teen Pregnancy, and HIV/AIDS* (Coyle, et al, 1996; Kirby, 2007).

Most parents support providing young people accurate sex education in schools, including reproductive science and methods of contraception. However, there remains some concern that if health educators teach methods for having safe sex, they will inadvertently encourage young people to be sexually active. Recent research concerning the impact of these programs is very important for resolving this controversial issue. In his review of the most rigorously evaluated comprehensive programs, Kirby found that, "Studies clearly demonstrate that the same programs can both delay sex and increase use of condoms or other forms of contraception. In other words, emphasizing abstinence and the use of protection for those who do not have sex in the same program is not confusing to young people; rather it is realistic and effective" (Kirby, 2007, p. 123).

If there is now compelling evidence that there is no negative impact of comprehensive pregnancy and HIV/STD prevention efforts, there is also growing agreement among scholars that few programs show highly significant impact on adolescents' sexual behavior. Kirby (2007) estimates that on average, the most effective programs reduce risky sexual behavior by about one third. While many programs are successful at increasing participants' levels of knowledge and skills necessary to reduce high-risk sexual behavior, fewer are able to influence teens to change their behavior accordingly. Nevertheless, within the context of modest findings, many programs do help teens delay sexual initiation, increase sexually active teens' use of birth control in general and condoms, reduce the number of sexual partners, and avoid pregnancy and STIs (Brindis and Philiber, 2003). Overall, these programs are effective with diverse youth in different setting such as schools, community-based organizations and clinics.

The most effective sexuality and HIV/STD education programs share certain characteristics of their structure, content, and method. The following section identifies common features of programs that have been found from rigorous evaluation to have positive impact on teens' sexual risk-taking behaviors and specifies practice implications. Effective programs:

1. **Focus on one or more sexual behaviors that lead to unintended pregnancy or HIV/STD infection.** Practice implication: Rather than covering such broad issues as dating or gender roles, emphasize a limited number of concrete behaviors such as how to use contraceptives or to resist pressure to have sex.

2. **Are based on theoretical approaches that have been demonstrated to influence other health-related behavior and identify specific important sexual antecedents to be targeted**. Practice implication: Activities should be designed to address those antecedents identified by theories of high-risk behavior. Specifically, programs should provide accurate information; heighten perception of risk of HIV; teach the value of pregnancy-free and STI-free adolescence; encourage positive attitudes toward condoms; teach skills to act on the value; enhance confidence in the ability to refuse sex, use condoms and other choices that will reduce risk; provide social support for such behavior; and encourage communication with parents and other adults about sex and birth control.

3. **Deliver and consistently reinforce a clear message about abstaining from sexual activity and/or using**

condoms or other forms of contraception. Practice implication: Rather than present information about human sexuality and family planning in a value-neutral way, advocate explicitly for abstinence and/or contraception during sexual intercourse. These are not incompatible messages. It is not confusing to present a hierarchy of values: "It is best *not* to have sex as an unmarried teenager, but if you do, it is better to use birth control than have unprotected sex."

4. **Provide basic, accurate information about the risks of teen sexual activity and about ways to avoid intercourse or use methods of protection against pregnancy and STIs.** Practice implication: Give students enough information to accurately assess their personal risk and to avoid unprotected sex without overwhelming them with details.

5. **Include activities that address social pressures that influence sexual behavior.** Practice implication: Identify the sources of social pressure that lead to unprotected sex such as individual partners, peer attitudes toward birth control, and media messages. Acknowledge barriers to prevention such as discomfort about seeking birth control or wanting to please a boyfriend or girlfriend. Provide concrete behavioral strategies for resisting the pressure and overcoming barriers.

6. **Provide examples of and practice with communication, negotiations, and refusal skills.** Practice implication: Show participants specific ways to resist pressure and provide opportunity to rehearse those skills through group exercises such as role-plays and other experiential methods learning. It is important to increase youth's repertoires of skills and comfort applying them in real-life situations though practice.

7. **Employ teaching methods designed to involve participants and have them personalize the information.** Practice implications: Include activities that make the lessons immediately applicable to participants' everyday experience, such as going to buy condoms at a pharmacy or role-playing refusing to have sex.

8. **Incorporate behavioral goals, teaching methods, and materials that are appropriate to the age, sexual experience, and culture of the students.** Practice implications: Tailor programs to participants' developmental

level and to the particular risks posed by their socio-cultural environment. For example, teens in very high-risk environments need more intensive group support for abstinence as an acceptable norm than teens whose peers are less sexually active. In terms of developmental stages, interventions for early adolescents should be geared to concrete thinking, give boys and girls the same information, and address what makes good relation-ships. For middle adolescents, use of peer educators, safe opportunities for physical and emotional risk-taking, and encouraging parental involvement are effective. While late adolescents are more adult in their functioning, they should be included in outreach efforts directed at their recreational, religious, and work settings (National Campaign to Prevent Teen Pregnancy, 1999, p. 38).

9. **Have sufficient duration and intensity.** Practice impli-cation: Exposure to programs over a longer time and more often increases the impact of programs on participants. For example, formal curricula that last less than a total of 14 hours can be enhanced by facilitating some other kind of group experience such as using peer volunteers on an informal basis. It is important to maintain fidelity in implementing standardized curricula and other program elements.

10. **Cover topics in planned and logical order.** Practice implication: Because attitudes generally precede behav-ioral choices, increase adolescents' positive valuation of and intention to avoid pregnancy and STI first, then move to teaching knowledge and skills necessary to avoid them.

11. **Select teachers or peer leaders who believe in the program and then provide them with adequate training.** Practice implication: Make sure professional and peer leaders have substantial expertise in the knowledge and skills imparted by the curriculum. They should communicate strong commitment to the underlying message of the program (Kirby, 2001).

Reinforcement through redundancy of messages and activities is an integral aspect of demonstrably effective sexuality and HIV/STD education programs. The absence of any one of these features can diminish a program's impact. More successful programs develop activities incorporating cognitive, behavioral, and social influence theories in various types of learning experiences. They provide limited and focused information; teach specific skills and create structured opportunities for their mastery; and actively create a safe social environment that explicitly supports acting on the value of abstinence and/or contraception, thereby increasing motivation for compliance.

In addition to abstinence-only and more comprehensive sex and HIV/STD educational programs, a third type of service that addresses proximal psychosexual antecedents directly provides *reproductive health care* and/or *greater access to birth control*. These services are offered in quite different venues. They include settings whose primary function is health care, such as public or private family planning clinics like Planned Parenthood and Federation of America, private physicians' practices, as secondary services in school-based health centers and school-linked health centers to which students are referred.

Services in clinic-based programs focus on providing young people with reproductive health care, including STI testing and treatment, as well as family planning. Girls are overwhelmingly more likely than boys to seek such services. For example, less than 5% of Title X family planning clinic patients are men (Edmunds, Rink, & Zukoski, 2004). In contrast, recent estimates suggest that 40% of all girls, age 15–19, make one or more visits to a clinic or private medical provider for family planning services each year (Kirby, 2007).

Clinics usually do not simply offer birth control to adolescents. Increasingly, health care providers view contact with teens in clinics as an opportunity for active prevention education. Most publicly funded clinics counsel teens about abstinence and also encourage them to discuss their sexual health with their parents (Kirby, 2007). Many clinics use various instructional and counseling methods to increase teens' knowledge of and ability to avoid risky sexual behavior. These include the use of videos, individual sessions, provision of written materials, and even rehearsal of proper use of condoms. Because so many teens have sex without planning, more clinics are now also providing emergency contraception that is effective up to 72 hours after intercourse.

It is clear that easy access to both clinic and private medical care results in many adolescents receiving reproductive health services, thus increasing the potential to prevent both pregnancy and STIs. Despite strong evidence of use of these services, it is difficult to gauge their precise impact on how many pregnancies and illnesses are prevented. Nevertheless, we do know that, like sexuality education, medical services that provide birth control do not increase either sexual initiation or levels of sexual activity among young people. They do increase teens' possession of and likely use of birth control.

Reproductive health care is also available in numerous school-based and school-linked health clinics. There are over 1,000 health clinics and 300 condom-distribution programs nationwide in middle and high schools. They offer some combination of services such as gynecological examinations, contraceptive counseling, pregnancy testing, STI testing and treatment, and provision of prescription contraception and condoms. Like other clinic settings, they have the advantage of providing individualized care and contact with a knowledgeable adult. There is no consistent evidence that these school-based reproductive health services decrease rates of pregnancy or STI among students. There is, however, sufficient evidence to allay concerns that such services increase either sexual initiation or levels of activity: they do not. In addition, programs that intensively focus on prevention both through abstinence and use of birth control may increase students' use of contraception.

Health-related services that have the most positive impact on sexually active teens' use of birth control go beyond simply increasing access to contraception and address a broader range of psychosocial issues. They also provide individual and group counseling services, initiate open discussion of contraception, and advocate actively for the practice of safe sex and/or abstinence.

Reproductive health services, including family planning, have tended to be focused on women. However, with growing concern about HIV/STDs and the expectation that young men take greater responsibility for pregnancy prevention, many facilities are attempting to make their services more "male friendly." Some programs are succeeding at increasing young men's support of their partners' reproductive health needs and their own use of primarily condoms for birth control, and also attempting to heighten young men's sense of responsibility about fatherhood (Becker, 2000). To influence both young men's and women's sexual behavior, reproductive health services must engage their many sources of motivation for having sex and for making decisions about pregnancy prevention.

Wherever the programs are located, reproductive health services should:

1. Make services available without a long wait;
2. Make services easily accessible in their hours and physical location;
3. Ensure confidentiality;
4. Offer counseling after a negative pregnancy test;
5. Be "male-friendly";
6. Include youth development activities to enhance prevention impact;
7. Seek the advice of teens in designing services;
8. Know the reputation of the program among its client population (National Campaign to Prevent Teen Pregnancy, 1999, p. 13).

These guidelines are responsive to the typical developmental characteristics of adolescence and should be considered when designing such programs for youths regardless of their intensity of risk. That is, they are a universal type of youth service.

Finally, there is increasing interest in the potential for mass media campaigns to reduce teen pregnancy and HIV/STD. Some campaigns address sexual psychosexual factors by attempting to influence youths' attitudes and beliefs about early and unprotected sexual activity. However, some campaigns have other objectives such as increasing community awareness of teen pregnancy as a problem, promoting a specific program or service, or organizing change on an issue such as support for sexuality education or a youth development perspective (National Campaign to Prevent Teen Pregnancy, p. 102). In Maryland, the state-level Campaign for Our Children includes multimedia presentations that convey mutually reinforcing messages to parents ("talk to your teens about sex before they make you a grandparent") and young people ("you can go farther when you do not go all the way") (National Campaign to Prevent Teen Pregnancy, 1999, p. 110).

There is a small but growing body of research to provide theoretical or practical direction for pregnancy prevention public media campaigns. One recent study suggests that media messages directed toward high-risk inner city teenagers must "combat positive attitudes toward pregnancy, negative attitudes toward birth control, the perception of personal invulnerability, and emphasize the negative consequences of sexual intercourse" (Witte, 1997, p. 137). Based on the Extended Parallel Process Model (EPPM) emerging from theories of health risk reduction, Witte (1997) suggests using an approach that combines fear appeals with messages that instill a belief of self-efficacy in young people; that is, scaring them into wanting not to risk the negative consequences of unprotected sex while communicating that they have the ability to avoid them through their own efforts. Early findings from a recent study of the additional impact of an intensive media campaign to small group delivery of health promotion and sexual risk reduction curricula suggest a positive impact on black youth in poor urban communities (Vanable et al., in press).

Such campaigns generally are one component of a larger set of activities and services directed toward preventing teen pregnancy, and it is difficult to isolate their effects. Nevertheless, given the hypothesized negative impact of media in glamorizing and encouraging sex among young people, it makes sense to assume that media can be used to counter messages of popular culture. As teens seek more information from the Internet, we must examine closely both its current impact and use the Internet creatively as an integral type of communication medium.

Nonsexual Antecedents

The prevention approaches described above directly respond to young people's need for accurate reproductive information, social support for preventing unplanned pregnancy and STIs, and interpersonal skills necessary to achieve that goal by avoiding risky sexual behaviors. In contrast, a second major category of pregnancy prevention services focuses on the nonsexual or *distal antecedents* to early and unprotected sex and pregnancy. The major nonsexual antecedents include community and/or family poverty, detachment from school, and lack of closeness with parents or other significant adults. These are the same factors that increase young people's risks of other problem behaviors in addition to early and unprotected sex.

Programs that address this group of antecedents usually attempt to decrease teens' risk of pregnancy indirectly by expanding their perceptions of and access to educational and occupational opportunities. An underlying assumption of this type of intervention is that increasing young people's capacity to envision and achieve a brighter future will motivate them to avoid high-risk sexual activity and pregnancy in the present. These programs fall under the broad concept of "youth development" and include programs both for young children and adolescents.

Despite the congruence of the principles of *early childhood programs* with social work theory and values regarding human development, there is not strong evidence that programs for disadvantaged young children decrease their risk later of negative outcomes such as teen pregnancy. A noteworthy exception is the *Abecedarian Project* (Kirby, 2007). Evaluation of this program found that infants in low-income families who received full-time, year-round day care geared to child development performed better intellectually and academically throughout adolescence than youths in the control group. Program participants also delayed childbearing by more than a year. One explanation for the better childbearing results is the positive impact of differential educational achievement on adolescents' fertility. Unfortunately, we do not know whether the lack of conclusive evidence from other similar programs reflects the ineffectiveness of the interventions or the methodological challenges of isolating the impact of complex programs over a long period.

Youth Development Programs for Adolescents Youth development programs for adolescents are growing in number across the country and take a wide variety of forms. In its broadest sense, youth development refers to the process by which young people mature into physically and emotionally healthy individuals who are able to fulfill their many adult roles in society. Recently, practitioners and researchers across disciplines concerned with reducing poor youth outcomes have emphasized a more specific definition of youth development incorporating the concept of individual resilience with a strengths perspective. In this framework, healthy development depends on youths having sufficient and specific protective "assets" that exist in their families, communities, schools, and other social contexts. For example, the South Carolina Department of Health and Environmental Control Office of Youth Development describes enhancement of youth development as: ". . .a process that prepares young people to meet the challenges of adolescence and adulthood through a coordinated, progressive series of activities and experiences which help them to become socially, morally, emotionally, physically, and cognitively competent. . .It strives to help young people develop their inner resources and skills they need to cope with the pressures that might lead them to unhealthy and antisocial behaviors" (Carlton, 2001). A common thread throughout the youth development approach is emphasizing and nurturing young people's capacities for success rather than focusing on their "deficiencies." Youth development also means identifying youths themselves as valuable assets to their communities and the larger society, nurtured through, for example, youth leadership programs.

The Search Institute's widely cited list of community, organizational and family characteristics that protect and nurture young people is frequently used as a guide for designing youth development programs. These assets include the following: a safe environment in the community, school, and home; a caring neighborhood and schools; adults who value youth; adults other than parents who support youth; neighbors who take responsibility for monitoring young people's behavior; useful roles for youth in the community; opportunities for youth to engage in community service; positive adult role models; encouragement to do well by both parents and teachers; clear school and family rules regarding behavior; family involvement in schooling; family support and communication; positive role modeling by peers; and opportunities for youth to participate in religious activities, sports, and other youth programs (Benson, Scales, Hamilton, & Sesma, 2006).

Youth development programs of all stripes are "sponsored by schools, churches, community organizations, civic groups, and local and state government, and involve young people in recreation, theater, sports, community service, and religious activities, among others" (National Campaign to Prevent Teen Pregnancy, 1999, p. 15). Within this large class of multi-activity programs, many youth development programs emphasize either *service learning* or *vocational education* and *employment* as core elements. Of these two approaches, only programs that focus on service learning appear to be effective in reducing rates of teen pregnancy (Kirby, 2007).

According to the Resource Center for Adolescent Pregnancy Prevention, "Service learning is part of a youth development philosophy that promotes engaging youth in constructive activities that build on their strengths and interests. Youth development programs hold promise for reducing teen pregnancy because they attempt to increase teens [sic]'motivation to delay childbearing by providing positive alternatives and leadership opportunities" (Kirby, 2001, p. 1). Service learning programs typically require youths to provide community service as a volunteer or for credit as part of a school assignment. Program participants work in hospitals and nursing homes, act as peer tutors, clean up parks, participate in charity walkathons, and contribute in many other ways to their communities. In addition to the actual service component, most programs include a structured opportunity to reflect on their experiences through discussions or written assignments.

One of the more successful service learning programs is *Teen Outreach Program* (TOP) (Kirby, 2007). TOP is based on the theoretical assumption that, "a critical task of social development is establishing autonomy in social interactions while maintaining a sense of relatedness with important others" (Allen, Philliber, Herrling, & Kuperminc, 1997, p. 618). Consistent with this view, "Teen Outreach is a school-based program that involves young people in volunteer service in their communities. The program links this volunteer work to classroom-based, curriculum-guided group discussions on a wide range of issues, from family conflict to human growth and development. This combination of volunteer work and classroom discussion clearly has the potential to enhance students' sense of autonomy while maintaining a sense of relatedness with facilitators, other students, and adults at volunteer sites by placing students in a help-giving (as apposed to help-receiving) role" (Allen et al., p. 618). A recent evaluation found that high school students' rates of pregnancy and school failure were considerably lower during the year they participated. The positive impact of this program suggests two important lessons. First, it affirms the benefit of explicitly theory-based interventions. Second, it supports the wisdom of taking a broad, developmental view of adolescents' high-risk behavior.

A different type of successful youth development program is exemplified by the *Seattle Social Development Program* (Hawkins, Catalano, Kosterman, Abbott, & Hill 1999). This program was designed to increase low-income children's attachment to school by improving the quality of teachers' instruction and parents' skills. This long-term study found participating children had higher academic achievement and lower rates of problem behavior, including teen pregnancy.

Integrated Models The third major category of prevention programs includes those that address both sexual and non-sexual antecedents. These comprehensive programs generally target high-risk youths in poor communities whose vulnerabilities are social, emotional, physical and educational. That is, the risk factors span all levels of individual youths' environments. Evaluations of this type of program are few, but they show promise for reducing high-risk sexual behavior and pregnancy among disadvantaged young men and women.

Although comprehensive programs that are neither long lasting nor intensive can have some positive effect on outcomes such as frequency of sex and pregnancy rates, one program has emerged as a model for working with young people at highest risk in poor communities. Recent results from the rigorous study of the *Children's Aid Society-Carrera Program* (CAS-Carrera) in Harlem found that the pregnancy rate among girls in the program were one half that of girls in the control group. This is a stunning result in a field of practice that has long battled frustratingly modest impact on vulnerable populations of young people.

The CAS-Carrera program was developed in 1985 based on the perspective that, "Teen pregnancy and childbearing is symptomatic of deep problems such as poverty, institutionalized racism, poor housing, substandard health care, inadequate education, and limited career opportunities. . .The desire to live long, successful, and productive lives and to achieve mastery over life's many challenges are what produce a genuine delay in the onset of intercourse or in the conscientious and consistent use of contraception during intercourse" (Carrera, 1995, p. 16). Carrera further assumed that these attributes are enhanced in children if he or she:

> . . .has a stable and nurturing family life, characterized by an adult who: (1) believes that the teen is precious and capable of "going places"; (2) supports the teen in setting a realistic life agenda; (3) encourages the development of a hopeful sense of the future; (4) regularly reinforces the

notion that foregoing early pregnancy and child bearing will enhance life opportunities. (Carrera, 1995, p. 17)

Many overwhelmed and poor families in Harlem, as in other impoverished communities, are not able to provide these important assets. In an effort to provide what is not naturally occurring, the CAS-Carrera program has engaged in long-lasting and daily contact with youths and their families through the following program components:

1. The Job Club and Career Awareness Components
2. The Family Life and Sex Education Component
3. Medical and Health Services
4. Mental Health Services
5. The Academic Assessment and Homework Help Component
6. Self-Esteem Through the Performing Arts
7. The Lifetime Individual Sports Component (Carrera, 1995, p. 18)

These components together address personal and environmental antecedents far beyond providing information and skills directly related to sexual activity. They are designed to change disadvantaged youths' orientations to themselves, to the wider society, and to their future; to increase their capacity to function as independent and successful adults. Thus, the program attends to young people's needs for sufficient knowledge, skills, and motivation to develop broadly their individual potential.

Two other programs that are less intensive though relatively comprehensive have shown some positive impact on boys' high-risk behaviors including, but not limited to, unprotected sex. *Project AIM (Adult Identity Mentoring)* focuses on helping young people develop a view of themselves that balances realistic expectations of the challenges of adult professional roles with optimism for success. Male and female AIM participants reduced sexual activity in the short term, while boys maintained the changed over a year. Project AIM developed a general risk reduction social development curriculum for students in grades 5–8 and compared the impact of the curriculum to the addition of a school–community initiative. The comprehensive initiative that included support by and linkages among various school and community members significantly decreased violence-provoking behavior, delinquency substance use, and reduced risky sexual behavior among boys, though not girls.

A comprehensive approach is very costly in human and financial resources, but sets a standard of how to diminish the multiple and interconnected sources of risk for youths in the poorest communities. Simplistic interventions that do not address the deeper developmental needs of young people may have limited impact over a short period, but will do little to alter the course of a teen's capacity for long-term success in adulthood.

The above review of major types of pregnancy prevention approaches suggests that there are many ways to decrease teenage sexual risk-taking and pregnancy. No one approach works for all young people, and each community will benefit by a particular mix of programs and services directed toward the needs of its youth population. The following chapter presents a framework for developing pregnancy prevention services targeted to adolescents' needs and their community context.

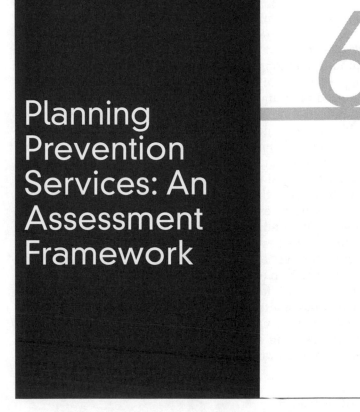

Planning Prevention Services: An Assessment Framework

As we saw in chapter 5, there are many approaches to decreasing teenagers' risk of pregnancy that are at least moderately successful. Given the multiplicity of potentially effective strategies, how should social workers decide on the best approach in any given service context? Decisions about program objectives and means of achieving them—the substance of the service—should emerge from a systematic process of assessing the youth population to be served, the organizational, the community, and the policy contexts.

Before discussing program development, a few qualifying observations are in order. It is not difficult, based on existing knowledge of human behavior, including the impact of planned professional interventions, to imagine an ideal prevention strategy that might dramatically increase any young person's ability to make healthy personal choices that

result in avoiding unplanned pregnancy or a sexually transmitted infections (STI). For those at greatest risk, such an
intervention would be very comprehensive in scope, intense
in contact, and long lasting. It would touch young people's
social and personal environments even beyond the reach of
such good programs as the Children's Aid Society-Carrera
(CAS-Carrera) program described earlier. The interventions
would involve structural changes through social and economic policy that improves public education, provides better
economic opportunity, increases access to health care, and
maintains physical safety for all children.

It should be a given that social workers collectively strive
to achieve these general social conditions. At the same time
that we keep in mind this broad vision, our attention must
also be directed to defining concrete, circumscribed, and
specific objectives for each program that promise observable
positive impact on our clients. This means carefully identifying realistic goals for behaviors that are actually changeable
with methods of intervention that closely respond to the conditions that influence those behaviors. Such a process rests
on sound assessment, as with any responsible professional
practice in social work.

Logic Models

The framework for assessment suggested here begins with
and expands on the key elements of a *logic model* used to
design programs and evaluate how well they achieve their
objectives. Though different types of logic models vary in
their language and elements, prevention program logic models should serve as "...graphic descriptions that show clearly
and concisely the causal mechanisms through which specific interventions can affect behavior and thereby achieve a
health goal" (Kirby, 2004, p. 2). In order to fulfill this important
function, the logic model minimally should specify "(a) the
health goal to be achieved, (b) the behaviors that need to be
changed to achieve a health goal, (c) the intervention determinants (i.e., the risk or protective factors) of each of those
behaviors, and (d) the intervention components to activities
designed to change each selected determinant" (Kirby, 2004,
p. 2). Figure 6.1 illustrates a generic model of the elements of
a teen pregnancy prevention program logic model.

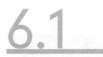

Elements of a Teen Pregnancy Prevention Program Logic Model

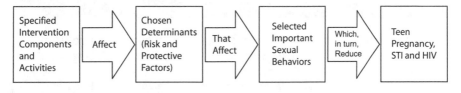

Source: (Figure adapted from Kirby, 2004)

Constructing a logic model begins with identifying the overall goals for the program and working "backward" to the program elements or activities designed to achieve those goals. Exhibit 6.1 is an example of a basic logic model for an abstinence-only prevention program in a school. According to this model, the program's goal is to reduce the incidence of pregnancy among students in the school. The target behaviors chosen to achieve the goal of pregnancy prevention are reducing the level of sexual activity and delaying initiation of sex among program participants. The program addresses a small number of individual (proximal/sexual psychosocial) antecedents that make sense for nonsexually active youth whose risk is low: instilling positive attitudes toward abstinence, decreasing permissive attitudes toward premarital sex, increasing clients' perceptions that their peers are not all sexually active, and increasing their perceptions that many peers favor abstinence. Four types of activities are chosen to change the antecedent conditions (individual attitudes and beliefs) that affect the incidence of target behaviors: group discussions, teaching interpersonal skills, peer involvement in group discussions, and student-led, school-wide events. Any number of other activities might be chosen in addition to or instead of these, depending on the service context.

Logic models of various forms are used across the social sciences and applied disciplines. Regardless of the particular format, the process of developing a logic model is highly consistent with the tenets of empirically- or evidence-based practice (EBP) in social work. Debate continues over the philosophical, ethical, and practical virtues and limitations of EBP for social work practice (Witkin & Harrison, 2001). Despite legitimate

Exhibit

6.1 Example of Basic Logic Model for Abstinence-Only Teen Pregnancy Prevention Program

Curriculum Activities	Determinants (Individual)	Target Behaviors	Program Goals
Group discussions about physical and emotional disadvantages of premarital sex	Increase positive attitudes toward abstinence	Reduce sexual activity	Reduce incidence of pregnancy in the school population
Emphasize that only abstinence is the foolproof way to prevent pregnancy and STI	Decrease permissive attitudes toward premarital sex	Delay initiation of sex activity	
Teach methods of expressing affection without having sex	Increase perceptions that peers are not all sexually active and they favor abstinence	Delay initiation of sex	
Use peers to lead discussions of disadvantages of premarital sex			
Have students organize school-wide activities such as theater productions and media campaigns that support desirability of abstinence			

criticisms of narrowly construed empiricism as applied to practice, using a logic model increases the likelihood that interventions are based explicitly on relevant knowledge of human behavior, practice outcomes, and their hypothesized relationships derived from a theoretical base. Specification of the expected relationship between desired outcomes and the means of achieving them is especially helpful, as well as ethically responsible, in the context of immensely complex and multiple influences on youths' sexual behavior. As a pragmatic consideration, when grant proposals include some type of a logic model, it indicates to funding organizations that the grant seekers have a clear and well-grounded plan for the program and their resources.

Elements Of Assessment

The overall goals of pregnancy and STI prevention programs are just that: to prevent adolescents from conceiving and contracting STI. Beyond these common goals, prevention programs should be built on local knowledge about several elements of the particular context. These elements include the characteristics of the youth client population, the organization, the community, and public policies (Exhibit 6.2). The issues included here in each element of assessment are essential, but the list is by no means exhaustive; rather, the categories are suggestive of the many concerns to be addressed by program planners.

Exhibit
6.2   Elements of Assessment for Program Planning

Youth Characteristics	Organizational Context	Community Context	Policy Context
Target population and level of risk	Mission, goals, and objectives of host agency	Existing services Service needs (new and/or coordination)	Federal, state and local policies regarding:
Risk and protective factors	Staff and administrative capacity	Values, attitudes and beliefs of community stakeholders	reproductive health care, public welfare, and sexuality education
Proximal and/or distal antecedents	Resources for evaluation		
Environmental level of risk factors	Funding requirements		
Characteristics of sociocultural identity, gender, sexual identity, andother group-specific needs			

Target Youth Population

- Identification of target population: universal or according to type of risk
- What specific risk and protective factors are present
- Whether the major antecedents are primarily sexual (proximal) or nonsexual (distal)
- The environmental levels of the risk factors— community, neighborhood family, and/or individual
- Characteristics of sociocultural identity, gender, sexual identity, and other group-specific needs

The first and conceptually, most central information includes characteristics of the youths to be served (see Exhibit 6.2). Whether prevention services are planned in response to troubling rates of pregnancy and childbearing and/or STI in the community (however, "community" is defined), to unmet needs among an agency's clients, or as part of universal youth development, the lynchpin of program planning is the specific sources of risk that the young women and men face. How high is the level of risk among the target population? What specific risk and what protective factors exist? Are these antecedent conditions mainly sexual or nonsexual in nature? What is the environmental level of the major antecedents? Among these antecedent conditions, which are most amenable to change? By what methods?

The answers to these questions will significantly influence the program's proximate objectives and target behaviors. For example, in a school district with mainly low-risk students, the primary risk factors may be individuals' attitudes toward nonmarital sex and lack of knowledge of birth control and how sexually transmitted diseases are contracted and treated. This situation suggests a universal approach addressing common sexual psychosocial antecedents—attitudes and knowledge—among the general student population. The target behaviors might be increased knowledge of how to avoid STI and pregnancy and the skills necessary to defer sex or practice safe sex. In the same school district, there is also likely to be a population of young people who are poorly attached to school and already engaging in multiple high-risk behaviors such as use of drugs and/or alcohol. This subgroup of students might benefit from more broadly defined prevention services addressing not only sexual psychosocial factors but also their mental health and special educational needs. In addition to the universally directed knowledge and skills, these youths might be encouraged to reduce the number of sexual partners and unprotected sexual acts and receive screening for substance use, depression, and other risk-heightening conditions. Thus, even within the same school community, the needs for prevention services may vary according to which young people are defined as the target population and their level of risk.

Another important aspect of target youth characteristics centers on distinctive needs, based on their race, ethnicity and other sociocultural identities, gender, sexual orientation, and other salient categories of diversity that may systematically influence the risks adolescents experience (Masters, Beadnell, & Hoppe, 2008; U C ANR Latina/o Teen Pregnancy Prevention Workgroup, 2004) Designing prevention that is, in its broadest sense, culturally competent involves attention to two conceptually distinct features: the methods used to encourage behavior change, such as didactic versus experiential techniques; and the content imparted by the chosen methods. At this time, there is scant theory or empirical research to suggest best practices based on cultural and other identity-based characteristics, including whether and when such are even indicated, but, as the developing knowledge base suggests, are important area for further attention.

One of the major challenges in drawing valid conclusions about the relationship between prevention approaches and the various identities of young people (complicated by the fact that most individuals are members of more than one "group" that may exert influence on their risks and behaviors) is that although many individual studies of interventions include diverse samples, few provide in-depth analysis of the significance of, for example, race in their findings. They may report that a particular intervention was more successful with African American teens than with white teens or with boys than with girls; but comparisons across different programs make generalization, let alone explanatory theory, difficult.

Within the general literature on reducing sexual risk-taking, research on STI and HIV/AIDS prevention tends to be more theoretically based and explicit about the role of diverse identities than the pregnancy prevention literature. A recent comprehensive meta-analysis of HIV-prevention programs examined the major assumptions about behavior change across different groups of adults and youth. Based on findings from studies of 354 HIV-prevention programs and 99 control groups, the analysis revealed important information about the intersection between intervention techniques and selected client characteristics. When programs use "active" methods such as counseling, HIV testing, and experiential skill building, individuals younger than age 21 are best served by "select normative arguments, attitudinal arguments, (information), condom provision, and self-management skills training" (Albarracin, at al., 2005, p. 859). With active intervention methods, clients across race respond to select attitudinal arguments, information, and self-management skills training, but members of racial minorities benefit especially from the addition of behavioral skills arguments and HIV counseling and testing (Albarracin, et al., p. 859). In contrast, "passive" methods involve presenting material with minimal client participation. In this context, younger people's behavior is most influenced by "select normative arguments, attitudinal arguments, (information), and condom provision" (Albarracin, et al., 886); while behavioral skill arguments are more effective with members of minorities in contrast to "majority" clients who make more use of direct provision of condoms. Though there is little analogous literature focused on pregnancy prevention with this level of comparative specificity, the increasingly rigorous standards for evaluation in the field hold promise for the generation of such important knowledge.

There is a nascent literature that provides guidance on shaping content of prevention to the particular characteristics of youth, again, most notably their race or ethnicity and gender (Horner, Carey, Vanable, Salazar, Juzang, et al., 2008). For example, in response to the rapid increase in teen pregnancy and parenting among the general category of "Hispanic" adolescents (which unhelpfully includes youth whose backgrounds include culturally diverse countries of origin), more programs are attempting to incorporate cultural norms into prevention programs. The National Council of La Raza summarizes the overall message of this literature in suggesting that effective programs for Hispanic teens include, "recognizing and sensitively responding to cultural values regarding gender roles; for example, some Hispanic teen mothers might not immediately see the importance of becoming self-sufficient" (Johns, Moncloa, & Gong, 2000, p. 6). Other recommendations include being aware of issues related to recency of arrival to the U.S., actively involving families of teens, and supporting education aspirations given the particular challenges that Hispanic students face in school achievement. Another growing body of research on incorporating sociocultural content into programming finds strong evidence that video and other media-based HIV prevention with high-risk African American youth is more effective when the content is communicated by people and in colloquial language that mirrors their everyday cultural environment (Roye & Hudson, 2003; Wilson & Miller, 2003).

Although these examples of culture-specific practice highlight the importance of considering bona fide cultural patterns in practice, it is equally important to remember that heterogeneity exists within ethnic and racial groups based on such factors as socioeconomic status, geographical region, location on an urban–rural continuum, and family and individual differences, among many others.

In addition to the growing attention to race- and ethnicity-based culture in designing effective interventions, the particular needs of young men in preventing pregnancy and STI are now being addressed through the "male involvement movement" (Edmunds, Rink, & Zukoski, 2004, p. 19). The following are the general "core elements of male involvement" prevention programs that emerged from the past several years of research:

1. Create male-friendly clinical environments.
2. Use gender-neutral decorations in practice settings.
3. Provide diverse reading materials that appeal to men.
4. Acknowledge men for participating in programs.
5. Include male staff in programs and train them in male reproductive and sexual health issues.
6. Conduct outreach activities in schools, youth groups, after school programs, religious institutions, athletic events, recreational settings, "hang outs," and other communities settings.
7. Target advertisements for programs to men.
8. Provide culturally specific materials for men from diverse backgrounds (Edmunds et al., 2004, p. 10).

Exhibit

	Assessment of Youth Population		

Level of Risk	Antecedents (risk/ protective factors)	Environmental Level of Antecedents	Sexual/ Nonsexual antecedents
Low	Attitudes and beliefs about sex and birth control; cognitive development; early sexual maturation	Individual	Sexual (Proximal)
Moderate/ High	Above factors plus attachment to family, school, and religion; general risk-taking behavior; family	Individual Family Peer	Sexual (Proximal) Nonsexual (Distal)
Highest	characteristics; income level; history of sexual abuse	Comprehensive: Community Peer	Nonsexual/ Distal Sexual/
	Above factors plus community poverty and disorganization; long-term family poverty	Family Individual	Proximal

This brief review of examples of tailoring programs is not intended to be exhaustive, but rather suggests the need for careful, detailed, and comprehensive assessment of those youth who are potential target clients of a program's services. (see Exhibit 6.3).

Organizational Context of Service

■ Type of host agency or organization including mission, goals, and objectives
■ Staff and administrative capacity
■ Resources for evaluation
■ Funding requirements

Prevention services are developed within a particular organizational context and influenced by many factors specific to the organization. Several of these key factors must be considered as the program is being designed.

Prevention services may be added to an agency's existing program(s), function as a freestanding program, or incorporate both such as the *Illinois Subsequent Pregnancy Project* (ISPP) in Chicago. In either case, the services must be consistent with the mission, goals, and objectives of the organization sponsoring the program. Prevention of teen pregnancy and/or STI might be the goals of three quite different youth-serving organizations: a hospital-based adolescent reproductive health clinic, a community center serving disadvantaged youth, and a middle school. However, each prevention program will provide a distinct set of services to achieve the same ultimate ends—reduce high-risk sexual behavior and its consequences.

The first agency may aim to reduce sexual risk-taking directly by increasing teens' knowledge of human sexuality and dispensing birth control. The target outcomes might include increased use of birth control and reduced number of unprotected sexual acts. In contrast, the second agency might offer a comprehensive recreational, educational, and community service program intended to provide prevention knowledge and skills as well as increase youths' perceptions of future opportunity, create the opportunity to have a relationship with an adult mentor, and enhance their motivation to delay pregnancy. Although the program goals likely would include reduced incidence of early pregnancy, proximate objectives might reasonably include nonsexual antecedents, such as improving performance in and attachment to school as well as positive attitudes toward condom use. The third program might adopt a service-learning curriculum that is integrated into the overall educational structure or directed to high-risk students only. Each of these dissimilar approaches has potential to reduce the risk of pregnancy if directed toward the particular needs of its target population of youths.

When a prevention program is being developed within an existing agency, an important consideration is the capacity of staff to provide additional services. Is there currently enough staff to carry out the program's activities? Does the staff have the requisite expertise? Even if a standard curriculum is adopted, it may be necessary to adapt the content to the particular ethnic or cultural characteristics of the participants. Staff may thus have to increase their knowledge about the substance of the services as well as their expertise with culturally competent practice.

Increasingly, agencies must carry out a minimally rigorous evaluation as part of public, private, or nonprofit funding mandates. Implementing a credible evaluation may require additional financial and staff resources. Some federal agencies require that evaluations of programs they fund be carried out by individuals who are external to the agency, thus adding additional cost for those services. However, even if the evaluator is a staff member, there are other evaluation costs. These include computer hardware and software, staff time to provide detailed information about the program, and possibly technical assistance for faithful program implementation if a standardized set of curricula and activities are used. Although many program administrators and staff regard evaluation as a necessary evil to fulfill funding requirements, a good evaluation plan and evaluator can provide invaluable ongoing information to continually improve the quality of service.

The sources of funding may also have a material impact on the kinds of services that can be offered. For example, services funded under the Adolescent Family Life (AFL) Demonstration Projects must be abstinence only and use activities and curricula approved by the Office of Adolescent Pregnancy Prevention. Many pregnancy prevention services are funded by more than one categorical stream, combining, for example, drug abuse and school dropout prevention grants. In this situation, there may be multiple restrictions or requirements for program content that must be integrated or coordinated. Even nongovernment sources of support such as private foundations may be invested in a particular approach that reflects its organizational values or research interests. These are considerations that should both guide service design and decisions about what sources of funding to seek.

Community Resources and Culture

- Existing services
- Values, attitudes, and beliefs of community members

In addition to assessing the needs of the client population and the organizational context, it is necessary to be familiar with the community whose youths and families are being served. One of the first questions to answer is what programs and services are currently available to address teen pregnancy prevention. In some communities, there are adequate youth services but they are being duplicated or are not easily accessible. Consequently, the intervention that is most needed may be a mechanism for coordinating existing, rather than creating new services. Many states and local communities are investing in creating coalitions or collaboration among programs to make more efficient use of their limited resources. Although developing well-functioning collaboration sometimes entails resolving "turf" battles among existing organizations, the greater the base of community support for an overall goal, the more effective will be that community's prevention campaign.

If the need for new services is apparent, it is critical to design them with full awareness of the varied and possibly conflicting values, beliefs, and attitudes of community members about teen pregnancy and related issues, such as premarital sex and sex education. It is the ethical responsibility of social workers to be sensitive to community members' responses to these emotionally and morally charged questions. It is also true that without community support, a program can face forms of opposition that will threaten the success of even a theoretically sound prevention program.

Often, a compromise among community groups with different views is reached by endorsing various program types within an overall coordinated prevention campaign. For example, in Wisconsin, the details of the state-wide *Brighter Futures* initiative were developed by an executive subcommittee representing the state Department of Health and Family Services, the Department of Workforce Development, several churches, and the Abstinence Coalition, among others (Farber, 1999). Although these stakeholders came to the task with clearly different value positions, they were able to agree on the goal of reducing rates of pregnancy and births with a primary emphasis on abstinence and a secondary objective of preparing sexually active youth to have safe sex. They adopted a broad, statewide youth development approach that left room for a wide variety of programs suited to the preferences of each local community. The original initiative has developed into the current statewide comprehensive youth development program emerging from community-identified needs and priorities:

> *BFI communities determine the target group for projects based on local needs and available resources. Services range from educational outreach, positive youth development, primary prevention and early intervention (secondary prevention). The projects focus on multiple aspects of a young person's life versus a single risk factor. Projects may change from year to year based on emerging needs in the community, new community partnerships, and program performance by service providers. (http://dcf.wisconsin.gov/bfi/.0)*

There are many kinds of communities to consider. A community may be defined by geographical proximity, such as a neighborhood with physical boundaries. A community may be defined by membership in an institution such as a school, including staff, administration, parents, and students. Members of a community may be affiliated by virtue of their religion or cultural identity. All of these and other kinds of communities exist simultaneously and may have compelling interests in how teen pregnancy prevention is conceived and carried out. These interests may be identical, complementary, or competing. They must be acknowledged and addressed in the formative stages of program development.

Failure to gauge and engage communities can produce negative reactions ranging from active opposition to lack of participation of young people and families in program activities. For example, when an AFL-sponsored abstinence-only demonstration program in rural South Carolina was designed without adequately consulting local education and business leaders, social workers failed to learn that parents in this deeply impoverished town did not view teen pregnancy as one of the most serious problems facing their children. In addition, the social workers did not anticipate fully the impact of the marginal economic base that forced parents to travel long distances between work and home. So, although parents supported the program's overall goal and permitted their children to attend the after-school and summer activities, they neither participated in the planned parents' group nor reinforced the messages given in the program. This frustrating situation could have been avoided by meeting with key community members and conducting citizens' focus groups before designing the program. The National Campaign to Prevent Teen Pregnancy provides practical, step-by-step suggestions for working with communities to develop prevention strategies (National Campaign to Prevent Teen Pregnancy).

Policy Context

Federal, state, and local policies regarding

- Sexuality education
- Health care
- Public welfare

Beyond the individual, family, organizational, and local community environments, there are public policies that can mandate, prohibit, or significantly shape services directed toward pregnancy and STI prevention (Boonstra, 2000). Federal, state, or local policies influence prevention strategies by, for example, legally excluding certain content from sex education curricula, requiring that certain health services be available to youths, or defining eligibility of programs for public funds and of clients for services.

Since the 1960s, the federal government has increasingly been involved in supporting services in the area of teenage pregnancy, with alternating emphasis on services to pregnant and parenting teens and pregnancy prevention (for a detailed history of federal policy through the 1980s, see Maris Vinovskis' authoritative *An "Epidemic" of Adolescent Pregnancy*, 1988; Donovan, 1999). In 1997, the Department of Heath and Human Service initiated the National Strategy to Prevent Teen Pregnancy. The joint administrative and congressional directive was ". . . to demonstrate a cohesive approach to the challenges of teen pregnancy prevention, and specifically, to provide assurance that at least 25 percent of communities in the United States have teen pregnancy prevention programs in operation" (U.S. Department of Health and Human Services [DHHS], 2000, p. 2). The Strategy was based upon five "key principles":

- Parents and other adult mentors must play key roles in encouraging young adults to avoid early pregnancy and to stay in school.
- Abstinence and personal responsibility must be the primary messages of prevention programs.

■ Young people must be given clear connections and pathways to college or jobs that give them hope and a reason to stay in school and avoid pregnancy.

■ Public- and private-sector partners throughout communities—including parents, schools, business, media, health and human service providers, and religious organizations—must work together to develop a comprehensive strategy.

■ Real success requires a sustained commitment to the young person over a long period of time.

The Strategy emphasized partnership and collaboration among government agencies, organizations at all levels from neighborhood to national, religious institutions, and other entities involved in youth development activities to enhance integration of services and pooling resources (DHHS, 2000). Perhaps the best-known program developed under this recent initiative is the Girl Power! Campaign, begun in 1996 as a national public education campaign intended to empower girls ages 9–14.

Currently, three abstinence-until-marriage programs provide most of the federal funding for pregnancy prevention. In 1981, the *Adolescent Family Life Act* (AFLA) program was enacted as Title XX of the Public Health Service Act. This program is administered by the Office of Adolescent Pregnancy Programs and funds three areas: care demonstration programs for pregnant and parenting teens, prevention demonstration programs, and research projects. The shifting political and hence, financial fortunes of the AFLA over the past 2 decades reflect closely changes in public and legislators' attitudes toward teen pregnancy, its causes, and the favored means of prevention. The politically conservative basis for the program resulted in a suit against AFLA, *Bowen v. Kendrick,* 486 U.S. 589 (1988), claiming that it was "administered in a way that violated the Establishment Clause of the United States constitution (separation of church and state)" (Sexuality Information and Education Council of the United States [SIECUS], 2001). In 1993, the Department of Civil Justice and the Center for Reproductive Law and Policy reached an out-of-court settlement requiring AFLA-funded sexuality programs:

■ May not include religious references
■ Must be medically accurate

- Must respect the "principle of self-determination" of teenagers regarding contraceptive referrals
- Must not allow grantees to use church sanctuaries for their programs or to give presentations in parochial schools during school hours (SIECUS, 2001)

In fiscal year 2000, AFL programs received $13 million to "find effective means of reaching preadolescents and adolescents before they become sexually active in order to encourage them to abstain from sexual activity and other risky behaviors" (Government Accountability Office [GAO], 2006, p. 11).

Beginning in 1998, funds became available by the Personal Responsibility and Work Opportunity Reconciliation Act of 1996 to states to use at their discretion that is consistent with the abstinence-until-marriage guidelines. In 2000, Congress increased funding through the *Community-Based Abstinence Education* (CBAE) program, which "bypasses state governments and has provided steadily increasing funds directly to community-based organizations [including faith-based organizations]" (Raymond, et al., 2008, p. 45). Administered by the Administration for Children and Families (ACF), the CBAE is regarded as the most restrictive funding streams in that, "Under its provision, grantees *must* target adolescents ages 12 through and 18 and they *must* teach all components of the eight-point definition. Grantees cannot provide young people with positive information about contraception of safer-sex practices, even in other settings and with non-CBAE funds. . .'Sex education programs that promote the use of contraceptives are *not* eligible for funding'" (Keefe, 2007). Between 2001 and 2007, funding of CBAE rose from $20 million to $113 million.

The ACF also administers the third major funding stream for abstinence education, *The State Program*. Grants are awarded to states based on a formula comparing the proportion of their low-income children in relation to the total number of low-income children in all states. Under this program, states must match every $4 of federal money with $3 of nonfederal funds. States have allocated these funds to diverse grantees such such as community-based organizations, school boards, health departments, local coalitions and advocacy groups, research firms, as well as direct service programs.

Despite the increased availability of federal funding for abstinence education through these and other programs since 1997, more and more states are declining to seek funds that require adherence to the strict guidelines of abstinence-only-until-marriage policy. California never applied for the abstinence-only funds; Maine, Pennsylvania, and New Jersey refused this funding in 2004, 2005, and 2006, respectively; and as of this writing, since 2007, Colorado, Connecticut, Massachusetts, Montana, New York, Ohio, Rhode Island, Virginia, Wisconsin, and Wyoming have followed suit in ceasing to apply for federal funds tied to abstinence-only-until marriage strictures (Raymond, et al., 2008). The reasons for states deciding to forego these particular federal resources are complex, but common themes reflect concern over the lack of demonstrated effectiveness of the approach and questions about medical accuracy of materials, as well as public support for comprehensive sexuality education as a better way to protect young people from the risks of high-risk sexual behavior (Raymond, et al.).

The Centers for Disease Control and Prevention (CDC) is the federal agency responsible for "prevention and control of infectious and chronic diseases, including STDs" (GAO, 2006, p. 13). While the CDC does provide support for abstinence-only-until-marriage interventions, it also sponsors comprehensive education through state and local initiatives.

Reproductive Health Care. There are several policies related to reproduction and health care that directly affect pregnancy prevention and pregnancy-related services to adolescents. Federal health policies create guidelines that may ensure or constrain the possibility of providing certain types of reproductive health care, but state policies ultimately influence such issues as the conditions under which minors have access to many of those medical services.

At the federal level, a key program is *Title X* of the Public Health Service Act of 1970. Title X was designed to redress unequal access to birth control by especially low-income women. It was enacted with the primary purpose of providing family planning services nationwide (The Alan Guttmacher Institute [AGI], 2001). Although family planning services tend to be directed toward women—nearly 2 million women younger than age 20 were served in 2001—they are also available to men. However, only about 2% of clients in Title X family planning programs are men (Becker, 2000). Teenagers represent 28% of clients who seek contraceptive services at publicly supported clinics (Guttmacher Institute, 2008).

Currently, over 2,000 agencies provide family planning services at over 7,500 clinic sites nationwide with Title X funding. Despite the diverse funding bases of most Title X programs, all grantees must adhere to the standards of care defined by the program including open access to all women regardless of financial means or age. Federal law prohibits using Title X monies to provide abortions, but programs must offer pregnant women information about all forms of prenatal care and pregnancy resolutions. Clients who seek contraception must also be offered related preventive health services.

Title X-supported clinics have several policies that encourage adolescents to seek care (CWLA, 2008; Gold, 2001). Fees for minors are based on their own, not their family's income. All clients, including adolescents, receive confidential care. Clinics must encourage minors to talk with their parents but service is not contingent on parental notification.

The provision of subsidized family planning to adolescents under Title X has raised controversy among those who believe that it increases sexual activity among teenagers. Others, however, argue that the program's affordable and confidential reproductive health services have helped adolescents avoid approximately 2 million births and a similar number of abortions. Although it is difficult to know precisely how many pregnancies have been prevented by young people using reproductive health care services, certainly these services have contributed significantly to prevention, and reliable growing evidence suggests that they do not increase sexual activity.

Another federal source of funding for adolescents' reproductive health care is through the *Children's Health Insurance Program*, the Obama admistration's revision of the former *State Children's Health Insurance Program*. SCHIPCHIP was established by Congress in 1997 to increase health insurance coverage for children younger than age 19 in families whose incomes are under 200% of the federal poverty level (AGI, 2001). "Originally created in 1997, CHIP is Title XXI of the Social Security Act and is a state and federal partnership that targets uninsured children and pregnant women in families with incomes too high to qualify for most state Medicaid programs, but often too low to afford private coverage. Within Fedcral guidelines, each State determines the design of its individual CHIP program, including eligibility parameters, benefit packages, payment levels for coverage, and administrative procedures" (http://www.cms.hhs.gov/LowCostHealth InsFamChild/). In an effort to extend states' provision of these health care benefits:

> On February 4, 2009, President Obama signed the Children's Health Insurance Program Reauthorization Act (CHIPRA), which renews and expands coverage of the Children's Health Insurance Program (CHIP) from 7 million children to 11 million children. CHIP was previously known as the State Children's Health Insurance Program (SCHIP)... In addition to renewing the CHIP program, the new legislation makes it easier for certain groups to access CHIP health care, including uninsured children from families with higher incomes and uninsured low-income pregnant women. http://www.cms.hhs.gov/LowCostHealth InsFamChild/) State programs may provide insurance by expanding Medicaid programs, implementing a state-designed program not based on Medicaid or by combining both approaches. In states that opt for expanding Medicaid coverage, young people are eligible for gynecological care and, by statute, family planning services for "minors who can be considered to be sexually active" (AGI, 2001).

In states with non-Medicaid programs, there is a range of reproductive services offered. The Alan Guttmacher Institute reports that, "of the 29 approved state plans that had some state-designed component, 16 specifically indicated that family planning services and supplies would be covered, while most of the remaining plans indicated that the general category 'prenatal care and pre-pregnancy family planning services' would be covered" (AGI, 2001, p. 2).

An important area of policy that varies significantly by state and continues to be disputed is minors' legal access to reproductive health care, especially to contraception, prenatal care, and abortion. The continuing policy debate centers around the extent of parents' rights and responsibilities to make health care decisions for their children versus the deterrent effect on teenagers seeking reproductive health care if parents must be notified. In recent decades, states have expanded adolescents' legal authority to consent to health care related to sexual activity, substance abuse, and mental health care (AGI, 2008). However, some states restrict the conditions under which a minor may give consent without parental notification, especially for abortion and, to a lesser extent, for contraceptive services. In a recent review of state laws regarding minors' access to sexuality-related are, The Alan Guttmacher Institute found the following:

- Twenty-five states and the District of Columbia have laws or policies that explicitly give minors the authority to consent to contraceptive services.
- Twenty-eight states and the District of Columbia allow minors to place their children for adoption.
- Thirty states and the District of Columbia have laws or policies that specifically authorize a pregnant minor to obtain prenatal care and delivery services without parental consent or notification.
- All 50 states and the District of Columbia allow minors to consent to testing and treatment of STDs, including HIV (AGI, 2008).

(See Appendix A for specific state policies.)

Unlike the liberalization of minors' access in these areas, minors have quite restricted access to abortion in all states except Connecticut, Maine, and the District of Columbia. In 31 states, a minor must obtain parental consent or inform parents in order to obtain an abortion. Many states impose a mandatory waiting period or counseling before permitting a minor to obtain an abortion.

Though these widespread restrictions reflect, to some degree, public values, in nearly all states restrictions on minors' consent for sexuality-related health care may be circumvented through a judicial (or, in a few states, a physician's) bypass if notifying a parent might cause the youth harm. Mitigating conditions are recognized in the case of minors being emancipated by marriage. Many state courts have adopted a "mature minor" rule that allows a minor who is capable of understanding the nature and consequences of a proposed treatment to consent to medical treatment without notifying or obtaining permission from parents. It is crucial to be aware of the specific state laws governing requirements for parents' involvement in young peoples' care when designing program policies and practice strategies related to any aspect of reproductive health or psychosocial services.

Public Welfare. One of the four major objectives of the Temporary Assistance for Needy Families (TANF) program emerging from the welfare reform of 1996 was to "prevent and reduce the incidence of out-of-wedlock pregnancies" (AGI, 2001, p. 1). This objective reflected the widely held belief that Aid to Families with Dependent Children (AFDC) program inadvertently discouraged marriage and contributed to rising rates of illegitimacy among both teenagers and adults. Though teenage illegitimacy was not the singular focus, TANF contained incentives for states to reduce their rates of adolescent pregnancy with the following programs.

First, the Illegitimacy Bonus provision of the Personal Responsibility and Work Opportunity Reconciliation Act (PRWOA) awarded cash bonuses to those five states with the greatest decline in illegitimacy (measured by the ratio of out-of-wedlock births to total births) while maintaining the 1995 level of abortion among all women. After making several such awards per the legislation, the most recent TANF reauthorization

> . . .eliminated provisions for Federal loans, the High Performance Bonus and the Illegitimacy Reduction Bonus and replaced them with a $150 million-a-year research, demonstration, and technical assistance fund for competitive grants to strengthen family formation, promote healthy marriages, and support responsible fatherhood. The Deficit Reduction Act also expanded a State's ability to meet its maintenance-of-effort (MOE) requirement. A State may now count expenditures that provide certain non-assistance, pro-family activities to anyone, without regard to financial need or family composition, if the expenditure is reasonably calculated to prevent and reduce the incidence of out-of-wedlock births (TANF purpose three) or encourage the formation and maintenance of two-parent families (TANF purpose four). (Federal Register, 2008)

Second, the Minor Parent Provision requires that unmarried minor mothers, with some few exceptions, live at home or in another supervised setting and stay in school in order to receive welfare benefits. This requirement is intended to address the concern that some young women bear children in order to receive the financial means to live independently from their families. Teen mothers may be exempted from the requirement of living at home because of abuse, neglect, substance abuse, or other mitigating circumstances. Many states provide so-called second-chance homes for teens who then qualify for TANF.

Third, the bill provided additional federal funding of $50 million per year for abstinence education through the Maternal and Child Health block grant program known as Special Projects of Regional and National Significance (SPRANS). These funds are currently administered through ACF in the Department of Health and Human Services state program, described above.

Fourth, the law places priority on establishing paternity and enforcing child support obligations of absent parents. It also emphasizes greater involvement by men in teen pregnancy prevention programs, encouragement of male responsibility, and education about statutory rape (Sawhill & Hutchins, 2000).

Fifth, the legislation gives states great discretion in how they use the TANF block grant funds as long as the expenditures support one of the four purposes of the program. So far, states have used most of their TANF funds for work-related activities to enhance independence and for targeted family assistance. However, preventing adolescent pregnancy is highly consistent with all of the objectives because of the strong relationship between poverty and teenage childbearing. The Administration for Children and Families, which oversees TANF, defines allowable teen pregnancy prevention programs as those that provide services for teen parents, prepregnancy family planning, counseling, or classes that focus on teen pregnancy prevention, and media campaigns (Sawhill & Hutchins, 2000).

States vary in how they distribute TANF funds and in the prevention strategies for which they use the funds. Wisconsin's Brighter Futures was conceived as one strategy to meet the TANF objectives. In South Carolina, the state legislature created the County Grants Fund for Adolescent Pregnancy Prevention Initiatives, which disburses county block grants to be used at counties' discretion. Georgia created the Adolescent Health and Youth Development (AHYD) initiative. The AHYD targets the neediest counties and supports comprehensive teen centers, male involvement programs, and community partnerships. In Massachusetts,

TANF funds support a statewide system of second-chance homes for teen mothers. Arizona uses TANF money to supplement Title V abstinence money in a comprehensive abstinence-only program. The three components include widely available abstinence education, a statewide media campaign, and evaluation of the effort. Significant state flexibility means that TANF block grants represent a promising source of support for creative program development at the local level.

Education. The main arena of educational policy with direct bearing on teenage pregnancy prevention concerns sexuality education in public schools. Although currently federal policy favors abstinence-only education, it is at state and local levels that actual policies about sexuality education are determined. As such, policies differ widely across the country and implementation of local policies within individual schools is even more variable. Although typically social workers do not teach sexuality education in schools, policies regarding allowable content will influence prevention programs that are school based or even school linked to any degree. Thus, it is important to know the specific policies governing sexuality education and the sources of influence on policy development.

Across the country, the vast majority of public schools provide some form of sexuality education (Kaiser Family Foundation [KFF], 2000; Darroch, Landry, & Singh, 2000). Inclusion of sexuality education in public schools has increased modestly over the past decade and also occurs in lower grades. At the same time, the emphasis in the content has become more restricted as more school districts have adopted an abstinence-only or an abstinence-plus policy. About one-third of school districts have no policy about sex education and leave the decision to teachers or schools. Of the 69% of school districts that have a policy to teach sexuality education, 14% require a comprehensive approach with abstinence taught as one option; 51% teach abstinence as the preferred option and permit discussion of contraception as an effective means of preventing pregnancy and disease; and 35% teach abstinence as the only option until marriage with discussion of birth control limited to its shortcomings (see Figure 6.2).

There are clear regional patterns in policies. School districts in the Northeast and in urban and suburban

6.2

Shifts in Formal Sex Education: The proportion of teens receiving any information about birth control has declined, while the proportion receiving information only about abstinence has increased

% of teens aged 15–19

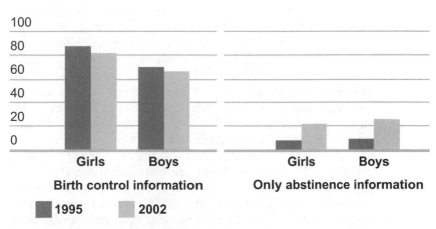

Source: (Guttmacher Institute, 2006, p. 2)

communities are most likely to have a district-wide policy to teach sexuality education. School districts in the Midwest and in nonmetropolitan counties most often leave policy decisions to individual schools or teachers. Districts in the South are nearly five times more likely than those in the Northeast to have an abstinence-only policy (Landry, Kaeser, & Richards, et al., 1999) (see *Appendix B* for state policies).

The increasing conservatism of policies has altered what is taught in classrooms: in 1999, 16% more sexuality teachers reported that abstinence was the most important message they wished to convey than in 1989 (Darroch, et al., 2000). Nevertheless, 58% of secondary schools have a "comprehensive" curriculum, and two-thirds of school districts permit some positive discussion of contraception.

There are many sources of influence on policies regulating sexuality education. Secondary school principals cite school district and local and state government as primary influences (KFF, 2001). About 31% report that the availability of federal abstinence-only funding has had an impact on their local policies. Within their communities, teachers, parents, community leaders, religious leaders, students, and local politicians are most involved in determining curriculum.

There are often disagreements among community stakeholders about the appropriate content of sexuality education. For example, there is a divergence between formal school policies and the preferences of parents in some communities. Recent surveys of parents nationwide show that, in addition to reinforcing an abstinence message, they overwhelmingly want sex education to include content on birth control, safer sex, and negotiation skills (KFF, 2001). In a recent example of diverse community members working together to influence sexuality education, the School Committee in Gloucester, MA held public hearings in October, 2008, that resulted in support for including comprehensive sexuality education.

The rising threat of STI and AIDS, as well as pregnancy, has certainly contributed to continued commitment to sexuality education in public schools around the country. Although abstinence surely is the most effective form of prevention of these outcomes, social workers must be careful to advocate for approaches that have the best chance of succeeding with young people according to their individual circumstances and needs. This often means facilitating negotiations among various groups of concerned citizens who may have equally genuine concern but very different preferences.

Summary

The assessment framework proposed here suggests a logical sequence in developing prevention programs that target specific groups of adolescents with close consideration of the multiple levels of the environmental context. The programming particulars will be determined by outcome objectives and will vary depending on the configuration of factors in the client population, the organizational, community, and the policy contexts. A clear rationale for choosing an approach and set of program activities will produce a better fit with clients' needs and heighten the chance of having a positive outcome. Youths whose risks are numerous exist at all levels of their sociocultural environments; they are both sexual and nonsexual and require a more comprehensive and holistic approach than those whose social environments provide strong support for healthy decision making and future achievement.

Few programs, especially those targeted to the highest-risk youths, can easily address the full range of antecedent factors. Rather, individual programs should realistically address a limited but well-defined set of objectives that follow from careful assessment of needs and existing services. This is not only pragmatic, but leads to more affective and efficient use of the limited human and financial resources facing all practice contexts.

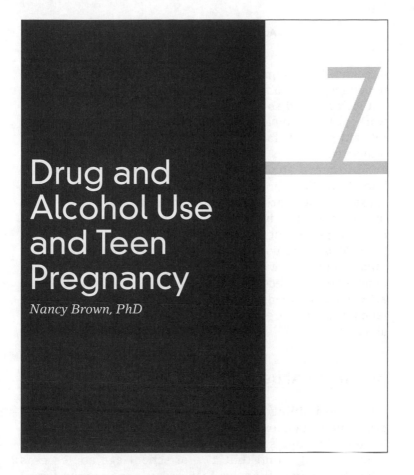

Drug and Alcohol Use and Teen Pregnancy

Nancy Brown, PhD

In 1979, I worked with pregnant teenagers at the Young Women's Christian Association (YWCA) in Schenectady, New York. At that time, Schenectady ranked among the top five cities in the state for rates of teen pregnancy. Interestingly, there was limited acknowledgment among community service providers of substance abuse as a problem for pregnant teens. Programs tended to focus on reduction of poverty, maintaining education, the prevention of second pregnancies, and parenting. Today, however, I can assure you that Schenectady no longer ignores the problem of prenatal substance abuse in teens.

Fetal alcohol syndrome was identified in 1973, but awareness of its implications in teenage pregnant girls took time to enter the practice consciousness. In the 1970s, teenagers occasionally reported that they smoked marijuana or acknowledged limited alcohol use, but this was relatively uncommon. It is obvious that you do not find what you do not look for, and so in the mid- to late 1970s, among social workers and medical personnel alike, the potential for a significant problem facing pregnant teenagers went virtually unnoticed.

Substance abuse among teenagers opens a Pandora's box of ancillary problems. Teenagers actively involved in substance abuse are significantly more likely to also engage in early sexual activity. Although teen pregnancy rates had been dropping, there was an uptick in the statistics from 2005–2006 along with even more worrying increase in the number of babies with low birth weight. With increasing evidence of the connection between substance abuse and sexual activity among teens, there is concern that today's pregnant teenagers are more likely to also be involved in substance abuse.

Substance Abuse And Teenage Pregnancy

Studies examining substance abuse rates and patterns of pregnant women are few, and even fewer for pregnant adolescents. Yet, one study (Kokotailo, Adger, Duggan, Repke, & Joffe, 1992) found that 17% of school-age adolescents attending a comprehensive teen pregnancy program tested positive for alcohol or other drug use. These rates are likely to be underestimated, particularly for those substances that are the most destructive. When comparing clinical identification of cigarettes to alcohol and other drugs, clinical providers were able to identify all cigarette smokers, but only half of the alcohol users and even fewer drug users (Kokotailo et al., 1992).

According to the 1999 National Household Survey on Drug Abuse, whereas 12.2% of pregnant women aged 26–44 years smoked cigarettes, 24.8% of pregnant teenagers smoked. Approximately 5% of young pregnant women (aged 15–25 years) engaged in binge drinking, whereas only 2.3% of women aged 26–44 did so (Substance Abuse and Mental Health Services Administration [SAMHSA], 2000). Young women, aged 15–25 (7.1%) were far more likely to use illicit drugs than their older counterparts (1.6%) (SAMHSA, 2000). The Centers for Disease Control (CDC) has noted that the rates of frequent drinking for pregnant women have increased substantially. The CDC findings indicate that the rate of frequent drinking among pregnant women increased fourfold between 1991 and 1995. Although drinking and drug use for pregnant women overall is about half that of non-pregnant women, it is pregnant teens who account for a significant portion of pregnant women who either smoke, drink, or use illicit drugs.

Substance abuse is strongly associated with early sexual activity (Smith, 1996) and drug or alcohol use often precedes the initiation of sexual activity by teenagers (Rosenbaum & Kandel, 1990). These statistics brings into focus the likelihood that today's pregnant teenagers will have a substance abuse history. It also suggests that today's pregnant teenagers have more problems that are of a more serious nature than ever before. Jessor and Jessor (1977) pointed out that adolescents with problems in one area are likely to have them in others. These problems are generally overlapping (Dryfoos, 1990), and the teenager is likely to have several of them at once.

The fact that pregnant adolescents are inundated by multiple problems is well documented (Dryfoos, 1990). Smith (1996) has pointed out that very young teens who initiate precocious sexual activity are at the highest risk for a multitude of problems, with teenage pregnancy and substance abuse among them. Smith (1996) notes that half of the teens who engage in early sexual activity become teenage parents. Although the number of women who use both alcohol and tobacco during pregnancy decreased during the 1980s and throughout the 1990s, this trend is not evident for younger women (CDC, 2000).

Several problems are cross-correlated with adolescent pregnancy and substance abuse such as childhood sexual victimization (Stevens-Simon and McAnarney, 1994), multiple sexually transmitted diseases (STDs) (Bragg, 1997), poor coping responses to stress (Amaro, Zuckerman, & Cabral, 1989), family alcoholism (Bragg, 1997), increased risk of human immunodeficiency virus (HIV) (Koniak-Griffin, Brecht, 1995), delinquency, school failure, and dropping out (Dryfoos, 1990). There are also many shared antecedents of substance abuse and pregnancy in adolescents. Genetics, family dynamics, developmental crises, and other psychosocial factors are all implicated in the initiation of substance abuse by teens.

Adolescent Substance Abuse

Statistics on adolescent substance abuse show complex trends. There are "cohort effects" which substantially complicate the picture for adolescent substance abuse trends (Johnston, O'Malley, Bachman, & Schulenberg, 2009). Different cohorts of high school grades reach peaks of use in different years creating unique and, at times, contradictory profiles for each group. In general, however, while drug use in the general population is down from almost epidemic proportions in the late 1970's and early 80's, and past year use has also decreased, drug use by youth ages 12–17 has remained relatively stable since a steep decline in use for most drugs in the late 1990's (Johnston, O'Malley, Bachman, & Schulenberg, 2009). Alcohol, cigarettes, and marijuana use account for most teenage substance abuse during pregnancy. By self-report, cigarettes are the most abused drug, with 17.8% of pregnant teens at an initial clinic visit reporting current use. Alcohol was used by 3.3% of the sample, marijuana 1.4%, and other drugs 2.8% (Kokotailo et al., 1992).

Alcohol and cigarettes have the most pronounced effect on pregnancy outcome, and it is important to take note of use and addiction statistics among teenage girls. Although rates of smoking have declined steadily since 1963 (Davis, Tellestrup, & Milham, 1990), the decline for teenage smoking has decelerated. Rates for teenagers remain steady, and rates for girls have continued to rise, and in fact, the rates of tobacco use among girls are now higher than those for boys (SAMHSA, 2000). Notable among the statistics is the fact that for African American youths, a group that had the lowest rates for decades, there has been an 80% increase in the rate of smoking, and that rate is rising three times as fast as the rate for white youth (CDC, 1998).

The percentage of teens who are likely to smoke one pack of cigarettes or more a day has increased. The suspicion is that those who could quit easily have already done so, leaving behind a group of teen smokers, more likely to be girls, who smoke more.

Although disapproval of illicit drug use appears to be increasing in the general population, the actual abuse of substances, including marijuana, remains stable for teenagers (NIDA, 2000). Marijuana is the most often abused illicit drug

(SAMHSA, 2000). The percentage of teens who report having used marijuana has doubled since 1991 (The Monitoring the Future Study, The University of Michigan, 2001). Marijuana use hit an all-time high in 1999 with nearly half of all 12th graders having tried it (49.7%). Use has remained basically unchanged, with 49% of all high school seniors having tried marijuana.

Cocaine and its derivative, crack cocaine, have been given significant attention by the media. In the 1980s and 1990s, cocaine and in particular its derivative, crack cocaine, were associated with media reports of catastrophic outcomes for babies born to crack-addicted mothers. Although later research did not substantiate the severity of the risk of prenatal cocaine exposure (Frank, Augustyn, Knight, Pell, & Zuckerman, 2001), the secondary effects of this drug addiction raise troubling concerns. Women addicted to crack cocaine are likely to be unable to provide adequate care, protection, or parenting to their infants and children. More recently, cocaine and crack cocaine have not had the intense media attention that was prevalent in the past. When attention is focused away from a drug, perception of risk tends to decrease. When perception of risk goes down, use goes up.

Ecstasy or methylenedioxymethamphetamine (MDMA) is a drug that has both stimulant and hallucinogenic effects. It has become popular among youth and is associated with rock concerts and large parties called "raves." Although the NSDUH began tracking the use of ecstasy in 1996, use of the drug has nearly doubled for high school seniors (6.1% in 1991, and 11.7% in 2001). At least one study has shown that ecstasy use during pregnancy is likely to result in brain damage for the developing fetus (SAMHSA, 2001).

Developmental Issues

Adolescence is synonymous with developmental turbulence. Teenagers who may have been good and compliant children can besiege their parents with a baffling array of behaviors. Stresses of adolescence are magnified in teens by their rapidly changing physiology, which precludes a smooth transition to adult roles and relationships. Adolescents look in the mirror and may feel that they don't measure up to peer expectations or unreal expectations. Those who are already negatively suffering from difficult life circumstances may also attempt to avoid pain or gather courage through the use of chemicals. These are also the same children who are likely to engage in early sexual activity.

Social learning theory suggests that teenagers locate multiple sources for modeling adult behavior in their environment, and with drug use is no exception (Bandura, 1977). They may first learn from and model their parents' alcohol and drug-using behavior. If their parents are substance abusers, drinking or using marijuana may not strike the adolescent as unusual or harmful. The second source for role modeling is the peer group, and it is no secret that pressures from this quarter can easily override any individual judgment process. If an adolescent's family, peer group, community, and/or neighborhood exhibit alcohol- or drug-abusing behavior, he or she may have little opportunity to avoid the pressure to experiment.

Women who abuse alcohol and drugs in adulthood are more likely to come from homes where substance abuse was prevalent (Nelson-Zlupko, Kauffman, & Dore, 1995). Young women who abuse substances are likely to have encountered multiple traumas or at least serious and personally threatening environmental stressors. These young women often come from families that also have a history of substance abuse problems, and they are more likely to suffer from several difficult, if not traumatic, experiences such as sexual and physical abuse, loss of a parent through desertion or death, rootlessness, and instability (Thompson & Kingree, 1998; Farrow et al., 1999).

Adolescent depression has been associated with family dysfunction, and adolescent substance abuse is a predictor of depression in adolescent women (Rao, Daley, & Hammen, 2000). Although the reverse is not true, it remains clear that there is a strong association between substance abuse, family dysfunction, and mental health problems in young women. Along with the association between substance abuse and early sexual activity, the case is made that teenagers who come from these families are more likely to get pregnant, and that their capacities for healthy pregnancies and adequate parenting are diminished by the magnitude of problems that they have and will continue to encounter. The circularity is astounding.

What Practitioners Need To Know

Social workers who work with substance abuse and teen pregnancy need to acquire knowledge in several areas. The first area is concerned with both the development and behavior of adolescents and issues of substance abuse. The second area that practitioners need to become familiar with is the association between adolescence, teen pregnancy, and substance abuse. Practitioners need to have an idea of the effects of different substances on pregnancy and developing fetuses. This includes how the physiological aspects of substance abuse are different for women and for adolescent girls. Lastly, the third area that practitioners need to be familiar with is issues of race, class, and gender because they relate to teen substance abuse and pregnancy.

Women and Addiction

In general, alcohol and drugs physiologically affect teenage girls in much the same way as adult women. Although patterns for adolescent girls have become more like their male counterparts in recent years, teenage women still share more characteristics with adult women than men (Toray, Coughlin, Vuchinich, & Patricelli, 1991). Social workers require knowledge about addiction as it concerns women in order to perceive the seriousness of risks for adolescent pregnant and parenting women.

Addicted women differ from men in three ways: physiological consequences, psychosocial factors, and patterns of drug use (Blume, 1992). When one examines these three areas, it is noticeable that the onset, course, and outcome for addiction are different in women. When looking at teens, we notice that there are also unique characteristics, and users of alcohol and other drugs do not represent a homogeneous group.

Social workers need to have a better understanding of biological issues, psychosocial processes, treatment issues, and political issues. In the 1970s and 1980s, research on women increased in response to the realization that there were differences between women and men in the use of substances. Use of alcohol and drugs and the subsequent addictive processes in teenage girls require an understanding of both women and adolescence.

Patterns of Drug and Alcohol Use

Drug and alcohol use by teenagers follows a pattern that be-gins with substances that are generally easier to obtain, such as alcohol and cigarettes. Adolescents generally do not start with drugs such as cocaine or heroin. Typically, cigarettes and alcohol are their first drugs and are considered by most researchers as being gateways for further substance abuse.

Adolescent patterns of alcohol use are often, but not always, different from those of adults. Teenagers are more likely to show a pattern of binge drinking. This may be a result of the sporadic availability of alcohol and the fear of getting caught. Patterns for adolescent girls are changing and, in some ways, are coming to resemble those of their male counterparts. However, because of the unique aspects of female metabolism of alcohol, teenage girls who drink are more likely to be much more intoxicated and have signifi-cantly higher blood alcohol levels than either teenage boys or adult men. They are also more likely to encounter the same types of problems associated with use as adult women.

Women's patterns of substance abuse are often associ-ated with stress. Losses, such as the breakup of a significant relationship, a job, or of social supports are often reported as associated with the initiation of substance use. Women are more likely to use alcohol and other drugs as the result of a specific traumatic event (Nelson-Zlupko et al., 1995). These events often include sexual abuse and physical abuse. Horrigan, Schroeder, and Schaffer (2000) refer to the "triad of substance abuse, violence, and depression" (p. 55). When one of these conditions is present in pregnancy, it is likely that the others are also present.

Women and teenage girls have higher rates of men-tal illness coexisting with a substance abuse disorder than their male counterparts. Suicide attempts, physical or sexual abuse, and family drug history are more prevalent among both women and teenage girls (Toray et al., 1991). So, while patterns of use may differ for teenage girls, overall they resemble those of adult females rather than their teenage male peers. Studies have shown that women in treatment for a substance abuse disorder are 30%–75% more likely to have been sexually abused (Root, 1989), and are likely to suffer from depression.

A sociological pattern often anecdotally remarked about by the workers at the Schenectady YWCA was the inter-changeability of the different groups of women who received services from the YWCA's various programs. When we went to the battered women's shelter to meet with pregnant and parenting teens to assess them for services, it was noticeable that many of the adult women in residence had, themselves, been pregnant during their teen years. Most were now in their 20s and 30s, and had returned to the shelter for issues of domestic violence. Pagliaro and Pagliaro (2000) note the association between pregnancy and domestic violence. This type of violence often begins during pregnancy and presents considerable risk to both the victim and the unborn fetus. Battery of this nature is also associated with the initiation of chemicals of abuse as a means to cope with the stress.

There is no protection for the developing fetus from sub-stances of abuse taken by the mother or by the risks encoun-tered in the social environment. The effects of substance abuse in pregnancy range from mild development delays and learning problems to serious congenital birth defects. The effects to the newborn are a consequence of the type and amount of a drug, the characteristic of the drug, and the general prenatal care of the mother (Cook, 1997).

Fetal alcohol effects (FAE) account for most of non-genetic birth and mild mental retardation in the United States. Cigarette smoking increases the risk of miscarriage and significantly lowers the birth weight of babies. Although our knowledge about the long-term effects of crack cocaine on the developing fetus has improved over the last 10 years, we still recognize that babies exposed to crack have serious problems at birth, even if they are not long term as was pre-viously thought.

Although the issues seem, at first, relatively easy to discern, substance abuse remains a complex problem with no simple answers. Compounding the risks associated with substance abuse are the risks of increased teenage sexual activity, particularly the high risk of contracting HIV and other sexually transmitted diseases. These, along with nega-tive outcomes associated with poverty, racism, sexism, and domestic violence, are woven into the environment of a pregnant teen and her developing child. These can't be eas-ily separated from the actual prenatal effects of chemicals.

Some things are clear, however. Substance abuse poses significant risk to developing fetuses and to the young women whose bodies nurture them.

Physiological and Prenatal Effects

Alcohol is the most serious of all the drugs taken by pregnant women. It is interesting that a drug that is legal at a minimum age has the most serious potential for harm to developing fetuses. Alcohol is embedded in the fabric of American life, and it has different functions within our society.

One drink for a woman raises her blood alcohol level higher than a man who consumes the same drink. There are several explanations for this. Men's bodies contain more muscle than fat, and muscle contains more water. Women generally weigh less than men and their bodies contain less water: their blood alcohol levels will climb more rapidly than their male counterparts. These factors contribute to women being more inebriated while consuming the same amount of alcohol. Also, men's stomachs contain higher levels of an enzyme called alcohol dehydrogenase, which begins the alcohol metabolism for men before the alcohol enters the blood stream. Because women lack significant quantities of this substance, given equal amounts of alcohol ingested, more alcohol enters a woman's bloodstream. Some researchers have suggested that hormonal differences also affect both the objective and subjective experiences of intoxication in women. These biological effects create special hazards for pregnant women and teens.

Women who are addicted to alcohol and drugs experience the negative effects of substance use sooner than their male counterparts, and have a higher mortality rate than men. This may be why women's addiction is known to "telescope"; women begin using drugs and alcohol later, but enter treatment at the same time as men (Nelson-Zlupko et al., 1995).

Alcohol is the preferred drug for teenagers, primarily because of the ease with which it can be obtained (Bragg, 1997). According to the 2006 Monitoring the Future Survey nearly 80% of high school seniors and two-thirds of 10th graders have experimented with alcohol. More than half of all high school students have had one or more drink within the last 30 days, and 46% of teens report drinking on a regular basis (Johnston, O'Malley et al., 2006).

High school students who reported drinking alcohol while in high school were an astounding 70% more likely to engage in early sexual activity (CASA, 2000). Although rohypnol, an amnestic drug often associated with date rape, has become a serious problem for young adult women, alcohol remains the drug most often significantly associated with sexual violence (CASA, 2000). The relationship between alcohol, teenage sex, and teen pregnancy is unquestionable.

Alcohol use has the most serious consequences for unborn fetuses. Fetal alcohol syndrome (FAS), a permanent disorder characterized by facial abnormalities, developmental and intellectual deficiencies in newborn infants, and fetal alcohol effects (FAE), the term given to babies who have a less serious form of FAS, are the leading causes of mental retardation in the United States (Van Wormer, 1995).

Although drinking habits for some teenage girls are changing and increasingly resembling those of teenage boys, the effect of these substances on their bodies is not the same as their male counterparts. Alcohol and drugs impact the health of women to a much more serious degree. With an increase in use by teenage women, these health risks will occur earlier and be more serious.

Nicotine and caffeine are central nervous system stimulants and are not necessarily considered drugs of abuse. However, they still have a negative impact on the developing fetus, not to mention the teenager herself. Nicotine has been shown to reduce birth weight significantly (Pagliaro & Pagliaro, 2000). Caffeine acts as an appetite suppressant and, along with smoking, also contributes to low birth weight in newborns. These factors are serious enough in themselves but may become even greater among teenagers who may not have good nutritional habits nor obtain early prenatal care.

Marijuana is the most abused illegal drug. It is generally either smoked or ingested by eating certain foods that contain it. Tetrahydrocannabinol (THC) is the active chemical responsible for the effect of marijuana. The subjective effects of marijuana include euphoria, an altered sense of time, problems with immediate recall, and increased appetite. Teenagers are often under the impression that marijuana does not represent serious drug use. Studies often conflict in their findings and this results in teens' unwillingness to accept the danger of marijuana. However, marijuana is illegal and, in many states, could result in the immediate removal of the newborn infant who tests positive for marijuana from the custody of a teenage mother.

For the developing fetus, the teratogenic effects of marijuana use appear to be low (Pagliaro & Pagliaro, 1996) and many studies show conflicting evidence of harm. However, marijuana crosses the placental barrier and has been implicated with lowered birth weight in some studies (Walling, 2001). Other studies have shown an increased risk of a rare form of childhood cancer (Walling, 2001). However, the evidence supporting marijuana's teratogenic effects remains inconclusive.

Inhalants are a class of drugs often abused by adolescents. These drugs produce vapors that are inhaled and result in extreme intoxication. Gasoline and glue are the inhalants most often abused by adolescents. This group of drugs also includes amyl nitrate, nitrous oxide, toluene, hair spray, and paint thinner. Overall, lifetime inhalant use is higher for the 18- to 25-year-old age group; however, past year use and current use of inhalants was highest for the 12- to 17-year-old group this year (SAMHSA, 1999). In 1999, solvents were the most abused drugs by 12-year olds (SAMHSA, 1999).

This method of drug abuse presents the most serious danger of severe damage to both a pregnant teen and her unborn fetus. Also known as "huffing," inhalation of these chemicals can result in sudden death cause by heart arrhythmia, which can occur from the first use (Espeland, 1997). Brain damage, lung dysfunction, and injury as a result of falls are also likely. There have been few studies that have examined the teratogenic effects of inhalants and solvents on developing fetus, but those that have been conducted find physiological anomalies similar to FAS and FAE (Pagliaro & Pagliaro, 2000). Because this group of drugs is abused most frequently by very young and middle teens, more studies on pregnancy outcome should be conducted.

Hallucinogens or psychedelics are often abused by teens. However, they do not seem to have significant teratogenic effects despite the folklore of the 1960s that widely reported psychedelics as damaging to deoxyribonucleic acid (DNA) resulting in fetal birth defects. There has not been any significant evidence of those effects. The physical and subjective effects include a rise in heart rate and blood pressure, hallucinations, and depersonalization. There is a serious risk for those individuals who have existing mental health problems. This group of drugs, which includes lysergic acid diethylamide (LSD), phencyclidine (PCP), and ketamine, can result in long-term chronic psychiatric problems (Fisher & Harrison, 2005).

Cocaine is a central nervous system stimulator. There are several routes of administration. It can be smoked, snorted, or used intravenously. Crack cocaine reaches the brain in mere seconds, and the effect is immediate. Cocaine activates the pleasure centers of the brain and bombards the receptors with neurotransmitters, primarily dopamine, associated with euphoria. It blocks reuptake of these substances, and continues to do so until the brain is depleted of the neurotransmitters responsible for feeling a sense of well-being (Abadinsky, 1996). As a result a "crash" occurs, which increases the likelihood that the individual will seek a return to the pleasurable state through the use of more cocaine.

Women who are addicted to crack cocaine are more likely to engage in high-risk sexual practices, increasing both the odds of pregnancy and of contracting a sexually transmitted disease (Inciardi, Lockwood, & Potttieger 1992; Greenberg, Singh, Htoo, & Schultz, 1991). When pregnant, women who use any form of cocaine may risk miscarriage, low birth weight, premature delivery, neonatal seizures, neonatal tachycardia, intrauterine growth retardation, and anomalies of the genitourinary system (Pagliaro & Pagliaro, 2000). Research reports of the teratogesis of cocaine have been controversial. Early studies showed severe adverse effects, but later studies failed to duplicate those results (Humphries, 1999).

Racial differences have been at the heart of the controversy surrounding crack cocaine. Crack cocaine use has been associated in the media and in research with women of color. Reports of "crack babies" and unrepentant "crack mothers" were portrayed in the media throughout the late 1980s to the mid-1990s. These mothers were predominantly black, poor, came from the country's most depressed areas, were uneducated, and were, and continue to be, victims of racial and ethnic oppression. Although the numbers of teenagers who abuse crack cocaine are few, the fact that the problem is associated with women of color warrants its inclusion in this chapter. Because of media attention and the political expediency of choosing the most vulnerable group (black, inner city, poor women), a criminal (in)justice approach has resulted in the nearly singular pursuit of crack cocaine-addicted black pregnant women, resulting in incarceration instead of treatment.

Assessment And Treatment

The assessment and treatment of adolescent substance abusers presents unique challenges to professionals. When the adolescents who are abusing drugs or alcohol are pregnant and/or parenting teens, the problems are even more complex. Symptoms of teenage substance abuse are typically different than those of adults. Adolescents do not ordinarily develop the same physical problems associated with long-term abuse. The social work practitioner has to look in other areas, generally more subtle ones, to assess the substance abuse problems of teens. When substance abuse is identified, treatment should be made quickly available and easy to access.

Identification of adolescents who are developing problems with drugs or alcohol is often compounded by the fact that many of the signs and symptoms of substance abuse are also those of normal adolescence. Risk taking, defiance, withdrawal from family, and increased reliance on peers is a normal adolescent signature. The problem is further complicated by the fact that definitions of substance use and abuse are wide ranging and not uniform. On one end of the spectrum, the National Council of Family and Juvenile Court Judges (1987) defines any use of drugs or alcohol by teens as abuse; at the other end, some believe that the label "abuse" of alcohol and other drugs can only be applied when there is evidence that the individual's use has led to negative consequences (Abadinsky, 1997). Thus, substance use can be characterized as a normal part of adolescent behavior (Trad, 1993).

Substance abuse and early sexual activity share a common etiological base: school problems, single-parent families, and childhood abuse, to name a few. Poor parenting and parental conflict, often associated with substance abuse by the parents, are more likely to be found in the families of teens with substance abuse problems (Jenson, Howard, & Yaffe, 1995). So many negative family factors are associated with teenage substance abuse that it becomes impossible to determine whether many of these factors are the cause or the outcome of adolescent and family substance abuse.

A guiding principle for practitioners is the understanding that no use of drugs, alcohol, or cigarettes is safe during pregnancy, and all use should be diagnostically indicated at a minimum as abuse. Identification of teens who are likely to be abusing drugs or alcohol while pregnant is paramount. However, complicating this identification is that teenagers typically do not enter treatment as the result of a self-referral. More likely, they are referred by parents, juvenile justice personnel, a child welfare worker, or medical personnel (Muck et al., 2001). The challenge in accurage assessment is further compounded by the special challenges presented by adolescence as a developmental stage, the current methods of treatment for women who abuse drugs during pregnancy, and the lack of prevention programs available to pregnant or parenting teens or women.

Despite these obstacles to identification and treatment, adolescents who abuse substances can be identified at several intervention agencies such as prenatal care clinics, schools, police or probation personnel, and child welfare services. Unfortunately, treatment professionals generally apply the same diagnostic criteria to adolescent substance abuse as they do to adults. However, addiction in adolescents often has a different etiology, course, and outcome. Therefore, it is important to find successful ways to identify and treat pregnant adolescents with programs that account for adolescents' unique developmental status, their unique substance abuse patterns, and increase prenatal care that will result in positive birth outcomes.

Similar to with other substance abusers, teens tend to minimize the seriousness of their drug use, and lack the cognitive complexity required to examine future consequences for themselves and their developing fetuses. Because of this, they tend to under report their use, which may lead the practitioner to underrate the problem. Assessment and treatment are further hampered by our legal system, which has moved in a direction where the rights of women have become separated from the rights of the fetuses they carry. This has resulted in a punitive approach to addiction when coupled with pregnancy. Women and teens identifying any drug use during pregnancy risk separation at birth from their infants, or worse, incarceration for many years. South Carolina has successfully prosecuted women for charges of child abuse and neglect. These policies are typically enforced against women who use drugs, particularly crack cocaine, and result in arrests most often of African American women (Moon, 1998). All of this only reinforces the tendency of pregnant teens to underreport or hide their drug use.

The psychosocial history is essential in providing the social work practitioner with information that is likely to identify a substance abuse problem and lead to appropriate treatment. In dealing with adolescents, practitioners should consider psychosocial risk level rather than severity of substance abuse problem when determining the level of treatment (Latimer, Newcomb, Winters, & Stinchfield, 2000). Fisher and Harrison (1992) recommend that practitioners explore adolescent substance abuse by looking in areas such as behavior, social relationships, changes in activities, changing tastes in popular culture, increased need for money, or large unaccounted for sums of money.

Medical personnel are in an excellent position to recognize and take the first step toward intervention. However, many doctors and nurses do not feel qualified in judging substance abuse behaviors. In one study, less than 25% of the women attending a prenatal clinic recalled if the medical staff had inquired about their substance use (Veach, Sheld, et al., 1995). If intervention could occur earlier, especially in a medical setting where pregnant teens are more likely to be seen with some frequency, many of the most serious problems associated with maternal substance abuse could be avoided or ameliorated. Education of medical personnel is important to prevention efforts.

Assessment instruments are useful in determining the existence of a substance abuse problem and the extent of its severity. One such instrument, the Simple Screening Instrument for Alcohol and Other Drug Abuse (SSI-AOD), is a self-report questionnaire that can be used by physicians and other medical personnel to assess adolescents in the clinical setting (Knight, Goodman, Pulerwitz, & DuRant, 2000). Other instruments, such as the Michigan Alcoholism Screening Test (MAST) and the CAGE Questionnaire are useful but less appropriate for women and teens (Piazza, Martin, Dildine, 2000; Knight et al., 2000). Knight et al. recommend that screening for alcohol and other drug problems become part of routine medical office practice when evaluating adolescents.

Substance abuse in women and adolescents presents unique challenges to social workers, counselors, and health care professionals. With the recognition that a "one-size-fits-all" model is not always useful with certain groups, treatment professionals have attempted to find innovative ways to deal with special populations. Our knowledge of how adolescents fare in traditional treatment compared with women in general is limited (Farrow et al., 1998). Typically, information about treatment of adolescents is based on clinical modalities directed mainly at adults (Jenson et al., 1995; Muck et al., 2001). It is important to look beyond traditional models and continue to investigate and evaluate new models for treatment of adolescent substance abuse.

Although efforts have been made in the area of adolescent treatment, there remain significantly less opportunities for pregnant women, let alone single pregnant teens or parenting teens (Howell, Heiser, & Harrington, 1999). Substance abuse is associated with negative factors occurring in women's lives such as poverty, abuse, and substance abuse by other family members (Howell, Heiser, & Harrington, 1999). In many places, the system actually discourages pregnant women who are locked in a cycle of drug and domestic abuse from seeking help. In South Carolina, the state now maintains institutionalized policy of criminalizing drug use by pregnant and parenting women. *Addiction* by definition means that an individual is unlikely to be able to stop a behavior on his or her own initiative. Research has shown that mothers who abuse substances attempt to cut down or do cut down their alcohol and/or drug use during pregnancy. Because of that first step on the part of the mother, this is a time when intervention is more likely to be effective. If identification of a drug abuse problem leads to incarceration, then fewer mothers, including teenagers, will seek prenatal care.

Treatment for women in most communities is likely to reflect the generalist model of treatment practiced in the United States today. Based on the Twelve Steps of Alcoholics Anonymous and Narcotics Anonymous, the generalist model offers group support, group therapy, and lifelong support for abstinence. Although it has been the standard for treatment, there is evidence that this model is less useful for certain groups, women and adolescents among them. Pregnant teens with substance abuse problems present an even larger challenge to counselors and medical professionals alike. Although pregnant, the adolescent remains developmentally in the same place as her peers, struggling with identity and questing for autonomy. Being pregnant does not advance the achievement of adult status; in fact, it is more likely to hinder it. Professionals treating the pregnant adolescent must accept the teenager as the primary client and must provide services based on a mutually respectful therapeutic relationship. It is often very challenging when the adolescent herself may not appear to be duly cooperative. However, social workers and health care professionals have to recognize that what they see is not always what lies beneath the surface. Pregnant teenagers will care about the outcome of their pregnancy, and substance abusers will care about the well-being of their unborn.

We need to place resources where they are most effective in helping young families. Treatment programs for parenting teens are rare, and programs that are available for pregnant teens are often concerned with issues of liability. Teenagers who are substance abusers will avoid prenatal care when they are threatened with criminal prosecution. With the number of publicized infant deaths attributed to teen mothers who have abandoned or murdered their babies, there can be no equivocating on policies that negatively impact a teen's access to prenatal care. Policies that result in arrest and incarceration of teen mothers based solely on substance abuse are not in the best interest of the infant, the mother, the teenage family, or society in general. However, models exist that are useful for adolescent women.

One promising modality is Multidimensional Family Therapy (MDFT) (Liddle, 1992). It has been used with success in dealing with teens with substance abuse problems, and incorporates elements that make it helpful to teens who are pregnant and/or parenting. In this model, teenage pregnancy and substance abuse are not viewed as unique or discrete events in the life of a teen, but rather are threads in a tapestry of factors that include the individual, family, and community (NIDA, 1998).

Effectiveness for family-based treatment has shown good results when compared with family drug education, adolescent group therapy, and individual counseling (Muck et al., 2001). Students who participated in a MDFT program improved their overall grade point average (Muck et al., 2001). This model, however, requires family involvement, which may not be easy for some teens, particularly those from families that are more destructive, chaotic, or involved in substance abuse.

Behavioral treatment models offer teens practicality by teaching specific skills that include communication, drug and alcohol resistance, problem solving, anger management, relaxation training, social network development, and leisure time management (Muck et al., 2001). Generally, this type of treatment can be completed in both inpatient and outpatient settings, as well as by an individual or within a group. Effectiveness studies for behavioral treatment models consistently show a reduction in severity of drug use, and the adolescents appeared to sustain those improvements over time (Muck et al., 2001).

Most popular programs for adolescents focus on a 12-step approach taken from Alcoholics Anonymous (AA) and Narcotics Anonymous (NA), both of which are considered to be self-help based. Through meetings and sponsorships, adolescents participate in a structured program based in the belief that addiction is a disease requiring management throughout one's life. The 12-step approach is often integrated into both clinical inpatient and outpatient treatment programs. Treatment programs typically utilize group therapy, individual counseling, lectures and psychoeducation, family counseling, written assignments, recreational activities, aftercare, as well as ongoing attendance at AA and NA meetings.

Studies regarding the effectiveness of 12-step programs have been mixed, but it appears that those teens completing programs based in the 12-step approach continued to do better than those who dropped out or those who did not enter treatment at all, at both 1 year and 2 years posttreatment evaluations (Muck et al., 2001). The 12-step programs often focus primarily on the drinking or drugging behavior of adolescents and do not address other problems typically associated with teen pregnancy, such as sexual and physical abuse or overall family dysfunction. This limited approach also creates issues for many women who are attempting recovery. Brown (2003) reported that women who have difficulty in early treatment often engage in high-risk behavior to avoid negative feelings associated with childhood trauma and abuse. It is likely that if the program does not deal with these issues directly, relapse rates among women will continue to be high.

Babor et al. (1991) suggest that it is also important to match adolescents to appropriate intervention levels based on degree of substance abuse, mental health, family and peer relationships, educational status, social skills, and delinquency. Additionally for pregnant teens, health status, pregnancy risk, and knowledge about parenting should also be part of the matching equation, along with the severity of other psychosocial factors such as family dysfunction, abuse and trauma history, and socioeconomic status.

Gender-specific treatment for pregnant teens has also been recommended (Hodgins, El-Guebaly, & Addington, 1997). Adult and teenage women are likely to have different needs in treatment than their male counterparts, and that is even truer for those who are pregnant or parenting. Programs that include comprehensive services addressing issues of substance abuse, pregnancy, and parenting skills are successful when working with adolescents who are pregnant and parenting (Uziel-Miller & Lyons, 2000). Substance abuse, pregnancy, parenting, sexual and physical trauma, as well as low socioeconomic status, sexism, racism, family dysfunction, and lower educational attainment status, need to be addressed to ensure successful lifelong outcomes. This holistic approach places a great deal of responsibility on social workers and treatment professionals to seek more complex and creative solutions.

Summary

The issues surrounding substance abuse and teen pregnancy are innumerable. There is the issue of harm to the developing fetus because of substance abuse of the mother. There is the issue of higher sexual and physical abuse among pregnant teenagers. There are also age and gender issues to be considered. Teen women are increasingly using substances like their male counterparts, yet they have more issues in common with adult women, both biologically and psychosocially. Poverty, sexism, racism, access to both prenatal care and substance abuse treatment, childcare, lower educational status, poor employability, and lack of health care insurance impact teen and adult women who are addicted far more critically than do their male counterparts.

The identification of women with substance abuse problems has often focused predominantly on African American and Latino women. These women, when identified by the medical system, are far more likely to be drug tested and to have their children removed from their custody than white women (Neuspiel, Zingman, Templeton, DiStabile, &

Drucker, 1993). This makes medical services and prenatal care a danger zone for any woman of color who uses alcohol and other drugs.

Knowing what do about pregnant teens who are abusing substances is complicated, yet our responsibilities and course of action are clear. Teens seriously involved with drugs or alcohol are likely to be poor parents, and likely to be at risk physically and socially. In fact, the social problems engendered in the lives of teens with substance abuse problems are often far worse than the physiological effects of consuming the substances themselves, condemning them to a cycle of poverty, sexual and domestic abuse, drug addiction, and social marginalization. Concurrent with these problems is the impact on the children of these teens. Not only will they suffer from the problems of the environment into which they are born, but the early bonding experience between a mother and her infant, an essential process for the best possible outcome for both teen and child, is placed at risk. When teens are separated from their infants, the bonding process can be damaged, sometimes permanently. Adolescents are concerned with external interests, and once freed from the demands of parenthood, they may find it more difficult to emotionally reconnect after a period of separation. Programs that maintain and foster these relationships, such as inpatient settings where the child resides with the mother during treatment, are the most effective in maintaining and supporting the maternal–child bond.

The key to successful intervention with teens with substance abuse problems requires flexibility in our approach to assessment and treatment. With the onset of the crack cocaine epidemic, we moved toward the practice of "remove the child first, ask questions later." Given the chaos that typically followed the life of the crack cocaine user, this was not unwarranted. However, with teenage mothers and the special problems they present, we need to expand our repertoire of responses. While protecting the infant in the present, we need to create processes that move them from a cycle of risk and abuse to an environment of support and guidance.

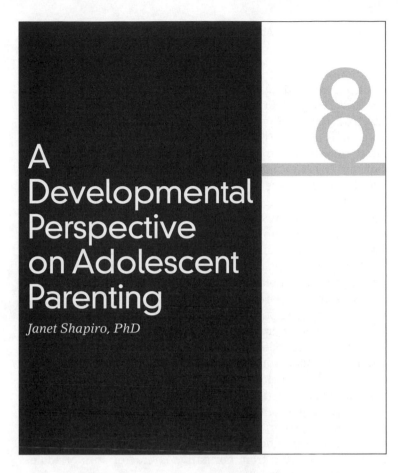

A Developmental Perspective on Adolescent Parenting

Janet Shapiro, PhD

Adolescent mothers and their children present a unique set of challenges to researchers, clinicians, and policy analysts interested in issues basic to the health and development of children and families. The developmental vulnerability of adolescent mothers and their children has been carefully documented (Cassidy, Zoccolillo, & Hughes, 1996; Furstenberg, Brooks-Gunn & Levine, 1990; Flanagan, McGrath, Meyer, & Garcia-Coll, 1995). A broad and multidisciplinary literature has resulted in an increased awareness of the developmental risks, for parent and child, associated with early childbearing and sustains our focus on adolescent parenting as an important social concern even as the birthrate among adolescents has continued to decline in recent years (Child Trends, 2001). The seriousness of these risks heightens the importance of sustained efforts to prevent adolescent pregnancy.

A substantial clinical and research literature on adolescent parenthood has emerged over the last several decades (Brooks-Gunn, & Furstenberg, 1986; Colleta & Gregg, 1981a, 1981b; Moore & Snyder, 1990; Shapiro & Mangesldorf, 1994). The focus of studies on adolescent parenting has shifted over time; broadening from a unique focus on the risks of early parenthood *to the adolescent* to the ways in which early childbearing poses risks not only for young mothers, but also to their children and extended families as well (Cox & Bithonely, 1995; Pope et al., 1993). Recent studies suggest that, although substantial variation in the quality of adaptation to early parenthood exists among adolescent mothers, the children of adolescents may be more uniformly at risk for developmental disturbance and delay (Shapiro & Mangelsdorf, 1994).

Recently, the parenting behavior of adolescent mothers has emerged as an important variable in the etiology of developmental delays observed in the children of adolescent mothers. As with mothers of all age groups, wide variation in parenting capacity exists among adolescent mothers. This chapter will focus on the developmental context of adolescent parenthood and examine the ways in which adolescent development creates a unique context for parenthood. This perspective supports a strengths orientation in work with adolescent mothers and their children because problems in parenting are viewed, in part, as deriving from normative characteristics of adolescent growth and development, as opposed to a singular focus on adolescent psychopathology. In addition, a focus on the developmental context of adolescent parenthood is important because it supports a conceptualization or risk and resiliency within this high-risk population of parents and children. This framework encourages researchers and practitioners to consider group differences between adolescent and older mothers, *and* important individual differences within the population of adolescent mothers and their children. These differences are not only of empirical interest; they are also relevant to the development of a range of primary, secondary, and tertiary interventions designed to promote competence among adolescent mothers and their children.

This chapter is organized into three sections. The first section is focused on historical and methodological issues in the study of adolescent parenthood. The second section of this chapter focuses on three sets of literature that may be combined to provide a conceptual foundation for the study of adolescent parenting as a mediating influence on the developmental well-being of children born to adolescent mothers. This literature includes research on (a) the importance of parenting behavior to child development, (b) the parenting behavior of adolescent mothers, and (c) the developmental outcomes observed in children of adolescent mothers. Lastly, the third section of this chapter will focus on development ecology of adolescent parenthood and the ways in which the developmental tasks of adolescence create a unique context for parenting and child development.

Historical and Methodological Issues in the Study of Adolescent Parenthood

The study of adolescent parenthood has been grounded in the assumption that early parenthood poses developmental risks to adolescents and their child(ren) and, thus, is a causal pathway by which young families accrue disadvantage (Brooks-Gunn, 1990). Flowing from this assumption are many descriptive studies that focus on the antecedents and consequences of early parenthood and on differences between adolescent mothers and those who delay childbearing (Furstenberg, Levine, Brooks-Gunn, 1991). Data from these studies are often utilized to inform the development of primary, secondary, and tertiary interventions designed to prevent or mediate the effects of early childbearing.

Early research on adolescent parenthood focused primarily on the risks posed by early motherhood *to the adolescent herself* (Clark, 1971). Over time, the focus of research on adolescent parenthood has broadened and has become more ecologically valid by addressing the impact of early parenthood on children born to adolescent mothers, on the extended family of the adolescent, and on the cost to society of early childbearing (Hofferth, 1987). In addition, early research on adolescent parenthood addressed the maternal age of adolescent mothers as a unique risk factor associated with a range of negative developmental outcomes for the adolescent. Research shows that maternal age is not a unique risk factor, but represents a more distal factor that is itself associated with a range of more variables associated with challenges to development (Ragozin, 1982). These factors include socioeconomic status, educational attainment, developmental immaturity, family stability, and marital status (Furstenberg et al., 1990; Hayes, 1987). Lastly, early research on adolescent parenthood was primarily descriptive in nature, focusing primarily on group differences between the children of adolescent and adult mothers. Over time, the focus of research became more process oriented, examining the pathways by which adolescent mothers and their children either incur developmental delay and disadvantage or are buffered from it (Fursteneberg et al., 1990; Shapiro & Mangelsdorf, 1994).

The above shifts in the literature on adolescent parenthood are important for several reasons. First, an increased focus on the social context of adolescent parenthood increases the ecological validity of research in this area, creating a more nuanced base of empirical understanding. Second, as the literature moved beyond a descriptive level of analysis to a process-oriented view of early parenthood, it became possible to develop models of risk and resiliency, differentiating levels of risk within this vulnerable population. This is of particular importance to practitioners who utilize this literature as a basis for the development and evaluation of a range of programmatic efforts.

Early studies on adolescent parenthood suffered from a range of methodological limitations. These included (a) poor sampling techniques and low sample sizes, (b) a lack of adequate comparison standards, (c) low ecological validity, and (d) a lack of multivariate analyses. More recent studies have begun to address these limitations (e.g., McAnarney et al., 1983; Whitman, Borkowski, Schellenbach, & Nath, 1987), and some researchers have undertaken important longitudinal efforts (Furstenberg and Brooks-Gunn, 1987; Furstenberg et al., 1990; Moore & Snyder, 1990) that offer initial opportunities to understand more about the life course of adolescent mothers and their children.

Studies that have examined patterns of individual differences in the adaptation of adolescent mothers and their children (Landy, 1984; Shapiro & Mangelsdorf, 1994) suggest that future research must continue to explore the heterogeneity of developmental risk within the population of adolescent mothers and their children. Some particular foci might include the quality of relationship existing between adolescent mothers and their children, the nature of adolescent mothers' support network and its influence on parenting and child development, and the adolescents' general psychological preparedness for the tasks inherent in parenting. This more nuanced approach to adolescent parenting will enhance our ability to form collaborative partnerships with adolescents and their families on behalf of the young children in their care.

A Conceptual Foundation for the Study of Adolescent Parenthood: The Application of Developmental Theory to Practice

Three sets of literature may be combined to support a focus on the parenting behavior of adolescent mothers as an important factor in the etiology of the developmental delays observed in children of adolescent mothers. First, a multidisciplinary set of studies demonstrate the correlation over time between parenting behavior, the quality of the parent–child relationship, and a range of social, physical, emotional, and cognitive developmental outcomes (Ainsworth, Blehar, Waters, & Wall, 1978; Schore, 1994; Shapiro & Applegate, 2000; Stern, 1985; Winnicott, 1965). Second, an accumulated literature documents differences in the parenting behavior of adolescent mothers compared with that of adult mothers who are matched on important contextual factors such a marital, educational, and socioeconomic status (Becker, 1987; Elster, McAnarney, & Lamb, 1983; Brooks-Gunn et al., 1986). And lastly are those studies that describe differentially negative outcomes for children of adolescent mothers as opposed to the developmental trajectories observed in children of older mothers. Each of these bodies of research is discussed below.

Parenting Behavior as a Mediator of Child Well-Being: A Multidisciplinary Perspective

From various theoretical perspectives, researchers have described the importance of parenting, or the caregiving context, as a determinant of child well-being (Ainsworth et al., 1978; Bowlby, 1969; Steele, Steele, Croft, & Fonagy, 1999; Stern, 1985; Winnicott, 1965). A rich multidisciplinary literature highlights the importance of parental behavior to a range of child development outcomes. This work includes studies from attachment theory (Ainsworth et al., 1978), early childhood education (Phillips & Shonkoff, 2001), and early social and emotional development (Schore, 1994; Shapiro & Applegate, 2000; Stern, 1985).

Research on attachment and, more generally, research on the quality of interaction between children and their caregivers, has expanded our understanding of the importance of positive early care. This knowledge base can help practitioners in assessing at-risk parent–child dyads and in providing more informed primary, secondary, and tertiary care (Shapiro, Shapiro, & Paret, 2001). The quality of caregiver–child interactions, sometimes indexed by a measurement of attachment security, is associated with a range of developmental outcomes in cognitive, social, physical, and emotional spheres of development (Cassidy & Shaver, 1999). Parenting behavior associated with secure attachment and with more optimal child outcomes is often characterized as warm, sensitive, contingently responsive, empathic, and attuned (Ainsworth et al., 1978; Stern, 1985).

The construct of *sensitivity* has been defined as the parent's ability to perceive and interpret the child's signals and intentions and to respond quickly and contingently (Ainsworth et al., 1978). Many factors may interfere with the capacity for sensitive parenting behavior. These include (a) lack of knowledge with regard to child development, (b) depression or other cognitive–affective disturbances that impair the parent's ability to interpret infant signals, (c) inability to put the needs of another ahead of one's own, (d) lack of identification with the maternal role, (e) unresolved conflicts over dependency, (f) high levels of stress, and (g) low levels of social support. Many of these factors are associated with adolescence and, thus, with the developmental capacity of adolescent mothers.

Researchers have developed models of parenting behavior in an effort to identify factors associated with variations in parenting competence (Belsky, 1984). Such models identify factors that either facilitate or impede optimal parenting behavior and, relatedly, child development outcomes. Generally speaking, process models of parenthood focus on three interrelated sets of factors that may combine to shape parenting behavior. These factors include (a) the psychological health and well-being of the parent, (b) structural sources of stress and support, and (c) a confluence of important child characteristics such as child health and neurophysiological status (Beckwith, 1990; Phillips & Shonkoff, 2001). Each of these sets of factors is considered in the broader context of the parent's own developmental history as well as in the social and ecological context of the individual adolescent, his or her family, and the community.

An underlying assumption of many process models of parenthood is that a parent should be an adult. Yet, adolescent mothers face the tasks and stresses of parenthood in unique social, psychological, economic, and developmental contexts (Garcia-Coll, Hoffman, & Oh, 1987; Shapiro & Mangelsdorf, 1994). As developmentally oriented researchers have long recognized, maturational differences between children and adults must be taken into account in the assessment and interpretation of behavior. Both adaptive and maladaptive behavior is best understood within a developmental context (Schamess, 1991). However, few studies have empirically examined models of adult parenthood in terms of their utility in predicting patterns of risk and resilience among adolescent mothers. Some of these studies have found that determinants of parenting competence among adolescents are patterned differently than would be predicted by existing models of adult parenting competence (Shapiro & Mangelsdorf, 1994). For example, increased social support (e.g., from the adolescent's mother) may not always be associated with increased parenting competence as one would expect to find among adult mothers.

The next section of this chapter will focus on development in adolescence and the ways in which the developmental tasks of adolescence may conflict with those of parenthood, creating a context for early development that may compromise the well-being of children born to adolescent mothers. This discussion is relevant to the consideration of (a) individual differences among adolescent mothers, (b) a range of assessment questions regarding the processes by which the children of adolescent mothers either incur, or are buffered from, developmental delay, and (c) the development of preventive interventions for this vulnerable population.

The Parenting Behavior of Adolescent Mothers

Research shows that behavioral differences exist between adolescent and older mothers (Becker, 1987; Hofferth, 1987; Levine, Garcia-Coll, & Oh, 1985; Hubbs-Tait, et al., 1996). The extent to which such group differences are found is mediated by many factors known to shape parenting behavior in both adolescent and adult mothers. These factors include socioeco-nomic status, marital status, level of educational attainment, psychosocial maturity, psychological health, the presence of negative life events, and the availability of social support. However, the pathways of influence between these factors (e.g., social support) and parenting behavior has been shown to differ between adolescent and adult mothers, as well as between younger and older adolescents (Landy, 1984; Shapiro & Mangesldorf, 1994). Thus, adult models of parenting com-petence may not be entirely descriptive of the experience of adolescent mothers and their children.

Compared with older mothers, adolescent mothers have been characterized as being less verbal in their interactions with their children, more controlling, less contingently respon-sive, and less sensitive (Brooks-Gunn & Furstenberg, 1986; DeCubas & Field, 1984; Elster et al., 1983; Hubbs-Tait, et al., 1996; Whitman et al., 1987). In addition, adolescent mothers are often characterized as expecting either "too much, too soon" or "too little, too late." Specifically, adolescent mothers are more likely to have unrealistically high expectations of their infants in the sphere of psychomotor development, as might be evi-denced by a young mother expecting a newborn infant to hold their own bottle. At the same time, adolescent mothers are also more likely to have unrealistically low expectations of their infants in terms of cognitive and linguistic development. For example, the observation that adolescent mothers are more likely to believe that an infant "cannot understand" speech, may explain why adolescent mothers have been observed to vocalize less to their children. This is important because research has shown that the degree of warm, verbal interac-tions at 6, 13, and 24 months is associated with measures of cognitive and social competence in toddlerhood. Likewise, an adolescent mother may be more likely to perceive an infant's cry as an indication of being "spoiled," which, in turn, may result in a lower degree of responsivity and emotional avail-ability, the two characteristics associated with many indicators of child well-being (Emde & Easterbooks, 1985.).

In summary, when maternal expectations of child develop-ment and behavior are based on false assumptions regarding normative development, they are likely to not be in synchrony with the child's capacities. Such dyssynchrony can lead to a cycle of inaccurate signal interpretation and subsequent paren-tal response patterns that are not attuned to the child's physical and emotional needs If such cycles of interaction begin, a parental sense of efficacy may be compromised (Greenberg, 1988). Alternatively, when a mother accurately reads and responds to her infant's cues, she is likely to get positive feedback regarding her maternal competence. This sense of competence is important to all parents, especially to very young parents whose sense of parental role identification is least societally supported and potentially most at risk (Schamess, 1990).

As with mothers of all age groups, wide variation exists among adolescent mothers with regard to parenting competence. Also as with adult parents, many factors are associated with variation in parental attitudes, beliefs, and behaviors (Sigel, 1985). The effect of maternal age on parenting capacity is more pronounced among younger adolescents (Landy, 1984; Shapiro & Mangelsdorf, 1994). Younger adolescents are more likely to display less acceptance of the maternal role, less cooperativeness and contingent responsivity, and less sensitivity in their perception of infant cues (Osofsky et al., 1996).

Developmental Outcomes of Children Born to Adolescent Mothers

Although substantial variation exists in the quality of adaptation among adolescent mothers to early parenthood, the children of adolescent mothers are more uniformly at risk (Brooks-Gunn, 1990; Moore & Snyder, 1990). Research on the children of adolescent mothers has paralleled the course of research on adolescent mothers themselves. Early research in this area focused primarily on the biological and/or medical consequences of early childbearing (Clark, 1971). Over time, the focus of research in this area has broadened to examine the impact of early motherhood on a range of developmental outcomes in the children born to adolescents (Elster et al., 1984; Field et al., 1980; Furstenberg & Brooks-Gunn, 1987; Shapiro & Mangelsdorf, 1994).

Compared with children of older mothers, children of adolescent mothers are at a disproportionate risk for (a) high rates of infant mortality and morbidity, (b) cognitive deficits and school failures, (c) child abuse, neglect, and entry into the child welfare system, (d) a range of social and emotional problems, (e) economic dependence, and (f) becoming adolescent parents themselves (Whitman et al., 1987; Brooks-Gunn et al., 1990). These effects decrease, but remain significant when contextual factors such as socioeconomic status, educational attainment, and marital status are controlled for in data analyses (Children's Defense Fund, 1985). In addition, the incidence of developmental delay in this population increases as development proceeds (Brooks-Gunn et al., 1990). Thus, the children of adolescent mothers are a population at risk for a range of negative outcomes and represent an important target population for primary, secondary, and tertiary intervention programs (Miller, Miceli, Whitman, & Borkowski, 1996).

Research on the effects of early parenthood on child development has focused more on a range of cognitive and educational outcomes than on the social and emotional development of children born to adolescent mothers. However, current developmental research highlights the relationship between socioemotional development and cognitive growth and capacity (Schore, 1994; Shapiro & Applegate, 2000). Thus, research that suggests deficits in cognitive development among children of adolescent mothers also raises important questions about the quality of the caregiving environment, the influence of a range of contextual factors such as poverty and social isolation, and the ways in which these factors exert developmental influence over time.

By elementary school, children of adolescent mothers are more likely to be described as distractible, disorganized, low in frustration tolerance, and impulsive. Such characteristics are often associated with being "unready to learn" and are associated with indicators of school failure such as grade retention (Brooks-Gunn & Furstenberg, 1986). However, as Moore and & Snyder (1990) point out, "there is a strong selectivity into adolescent parenthood, and even more so, into school failure" (p. 32). These researchers are highlighting the importance of factors such as antecedents to early parenthood itself and other variables such as maternal educational attainment and socioeconomic status that are also associated with cognitive development and academic achievement.

Research on the social and emotional development of children born to adolescent mothers suggests important areas for assessment and intervention in this at-risk population. Some studies have suggested that the children of adolescent mothers are less likely to be securely attached than are children of older mothers (Crockenberg, 1987; Hubbs-Tait, et al., 1996). Embedded within studies of attachment are a range of maternal behaviors, such as sensitivity and the capacity for empathic relatedness. Clinical researchers have observed that adolescent mothers face particular challenges, derived both from normative developmental issues and the presence of other risks, such as depression, in the regulation of affect and in sustaining empathic interaction with their children (Hubbs-Tait, et al., 1996). These findings are particularly important in light of recent research that describes the importance of early caregiving to brain development in early life and, relatedly, to the neurobiological substrate of a range of adaptive capacities (Siegel, 1999).

Studies of the caregiving context for children of adolescent mothers are complicated because the circle of care provided to the infant and young children often includes the adolescent mother, as well as grandparent care and/or the care of others in the extended family. The presence of a caring grandparent or other adult caregiver has been shown to buffer young children from some of the risk associated with adolescent parenthood (Colletta & Lee, 1983). Still, other research suggests that while the presence of grandparent care may be helpful in the short run, it may challenge the adolescent mother's identification with the maternal role, and thus interfere with the process of parent–child attachment (Brooks-Gunn et al., 1990). This conflict is an example of the dual developmental crisis associated with adolescent motherhood. One of the primary social challenges is finding a multigenerational solution that enables the adolescent to continue on an age-appropriate developmental track while at the same time, providing a developmental context for the young child that potentiates developmental growth and competence.

The Developmental Ecology of Adolescent Parenthood

The study of adolescent parenthood presents an opportunity to observe the superimposition of two developmental phases, adolescence and parenthood, that are usually temporally separated in our society. The developmental tasks of adolescence may conflict with those of parenthood, creating a compromised psychological context for the development of adolescent mothers and their children. It is in this sense that adolescent motherhood may precipitate a dual developmental crisis (Sadler & Catrone, 1983). For example, the normative adolescent behavior of experimenting with various roles in the process of identity formation may conflict with the parenting task of fixed maternal role identification (Mercer, 1986).

The idea of unresolved developmental conflict in parenthood is not new (Benedek, 1959; Fraiberg, 1980). In many models of adult parenthood, mastery over the developmental tasks of adolescence is understood as a predictor of parenting competence (Fraiberg, 1980). Among adult parents, it is "unresolved adolescent conflicts" which are thought to precipitate some of the most severe parent–child relational problems. When an adolescent mother's own developmental trajectory is interrupted by early or "off-timed" parenthood (the development of the adolescent's current and future parenting capacity may be impaired, creating an "at-risk" relational environment for the developing child.

In her early work on the adolescent experience of pregnancy, Hatcher (1976) noted that the "experience of any adolescent crisis, and especially one of a psychophysiological nature, is influenced by the developmental stage during which it happens to occur" (p. 408). Extending this argument to encompass not only pregnancy, but also parenthood, allows for the construction of hypotheses regarding the influence of normative adolescent development on the psychological experience of early parenthood, and the ways in which the normative tasks of adolescent development may conflict with the developmental tasks associated with parenthood. This view also reflects current understanding in models of developmental psychopathology that suggest that behavior, both functional and dysfunctional, must be understood within the context of normative development.

Mastery over the developmental tasks of adolescence requires the negotiation of stressful life events for all adolescents (Brooks-Gunn et al., 1990). Adolescent mothers must negotiate not only normative, age-related developmental transformations, but also the early acquisition of the maternal role (Kissman & Shapiro, 1990). Moreover, adolescent mothers are more likely to occupy a social ecology characterized by high levels of stress and low levels of personal, familial, and/or societal support. Together, these factors are associated with risks to parenting competence and pose risks to child development outcomes as well (Crockenberg, 1987).

The focus of the following section is on development in adolescence and the implications of developmental achievement in adolescence for parenting capacity. Further, this chapter will examine the ways in which adolescence, as a life phase, raises particular questions about the nature of social support, a factor identified as predictive of parenting competence and child well-being in many models of parenthood.

Development in Adolescence

Adolescence, as a life phase, has long been conceptualized as a period of rapid growth and adaptation along many developmental lines (Blos, 1962; Elkind, 1974; Freud, 1958; Hill, 1987). Despite differences of opinion as to the processes by which development occurs in adolescence, more general agreement exists regarding the major developmental tasks and achievements of this life phase.

Historically, *adolescence* has been defined by psychological, social, and maturational indices (Elder, 1980). Such indices of development are commonly utilized in "age or stage" or "epigenetic" models of development (Blos, 1962, 1962; Erikson, 1958). Social indices of adolescent development describe the timing and occurrence of life events (e.g., completion of schooling) and reflect important cohort variation in the expected timing of events (Elder, 1980) as is represented by expected timetables with regard to the transition to adulthood or parenthood.

Psychoanalytic theorists have long characterized adolescence as a "turbulent" period, one in which the individual experiences "inner turmoil," "storm and stress," and may manifest behavioral instability (Blos, 1962; Freud, 1958). According to psychoanalytic theory, the adolescent's developing ego must simultaneously accommodate the upsurge of instinctual drive activity precipitated by pubertal development and must manage increasing psychological separation from parental figures, relying less on the parental ego as an extension, or auxiliary support, of one's own (Hatcher, 1976). When seen from this perspective, development in adolescence creates a temporary psychological risk, or vulnerability, for adolescents because while in the process of differentiating from parental figures, they may not yet have developed important ego strengths and internalized coping abilities.

Other theorists challenge the traditional psychoanalytic view that adolescence is a time of universal upset (Offer & Offer, 1975). These researchers suggest that many pathways through adolescence are possible, and that not all adolescents experience the high degrees of psychological distress and turmoil. It is also important to recognize that although adolescents may experience a range of vulnerabilities during this life phase, other developmental lines move forward in ways that create new skills and capacities (Elkind, 1974). Specifically, adolescence is a time of growth with regard to cognitive development in ways that support new skills such as problem solving, the capacity for abstract thinking, and the ability to think about how one's choices and behavior may affect the future (Elkind, 1974; Most recently, developmental researchers have begun to articulate a more complex biopsychosocial model of adolescent development (Hill, 1987) in which the psychological, physiological, and social dimensions of this life phase are combined to form particularized matrices of development. Factors such as educational aptitude and achievement, social support and stress, economic opportunities and family stabiility are combined with indices of psychological well-being to particularize the adolescent experience for each individual. Further increasing the ecological validity of these models is the recognition of cultural and cohort variation with regard to the meaning of adolescence and expectations with regard to autonomous functioning in a range of spheres (Gibbs & Huang, 1999). Taken together, these factors are clearly relevant to understanding the ways in which the adolescent experience creates a unique context for pregnancy, parenthood, and child development.

The psychological "end" of adolescence is marked by mastery over a range of developmental tasks. These include (a) psychological separation and individuation from parents, (b) accommodation to adult physical characteristics and body image, (c) the synthesis and consolidation of a stable ego identity that provides the basis for personality integration across time, and (d) increases in cognitive complexity as evidenced in capacities for reality testing, judgment, self-reflection, abstraction, and future orientation. These achievements are in turn related to other strengths such as an increased capacity for autonomous functioning, increased ability for involvement in relationship and work commitments, and an increased capacity for the internal modulation of affect and self-esteem. Each of these achievements relates to parenting ability in important ways (Beckwith, 1990; Shapiro & Mangelsdorf, 1994).

Psychological Issues in the Study of Adolescent Development

Three psychological processes are often the focus of developmental and clinical research on adolescent development. These are (a) the nature of separation and individuation from one's family of origin, (b) the processes of identity formation, and (c) the emergence of increased cognitive complexity in adolescence. Each of these processes will be considered in this section in terms of their import for parenting capacity and will be revisited in the following section on the subphases of adolescent development.

Separation and Individuation

By naming adolescence the "second phase of separation and individuation," Blos (1967) drew a parallel between a primary developmental task of adolescence and the first phase of separation or individuation occurring at or around the end of the second year of life. In both phases, there exists a maturational push toward higher levels of autonomous functioning which requires (a) continued psychological change with regard to primary relationships, (b) adaptation to increased maturational demands, and (c) temporary vulnerability as tasks once shared between child and caregiver become more autonomous and require the integration of new capacities and coping skills.

Historically, psychoanalytic theorists have viewed the processes of separation and individuation as being intricately tied to the process of ego identity development. The process of ego identity development requires the adolescent to synthesize past identifications with current experience and maturational demands. Adequate progress in the processes of separation and individuation results in important structural changes in personality by the end of adolescence. Self and object representations acquire internal stability, no longer as dependent on external sources of validation, lending a constancy to self-esteem and the internal regulation of affective states. When adequate gains toward separation and individuation do not occur, ego functions that normally become solidified in adolescence, such as reality testing and the regulation of self-esteem, may remain overly dependent on external sources and thus, prone to regression under stress.

The developmental demands and social realities of parenthood may conflict with the tasks of separation and individuation. Normatively, increasing autonomy and reducing dependency are salient aspects of adolescent development. However, the acquisition of the parental role often heightens the adolescent mother's dependency on her family of origin. If this upsurge in dependency occurs in a psychological context in which the adolescent had hoped that becoming a mother would "make me an adult" or would "get me out from under" parental rules and authority, the dissonance between expectation and reality may precipitate feelings of disappointment, depression, and/or resentment. These feelings may be directed toward the adolescent's parent, herself, or more unhappily, toward the developing infant and young child. In these cases, resolving the adolescent's dependency conflicts in a way that promotes adaptation for both the adolescent mother and her child may require a multigenerational solution. The adolescent's own parent(s) may need support in understanding the adolescent's simultaneous need for and rejection of their assistance. Similarly, the adolescent mother may need assistance in coping with the continuous dependency needs of her own child. Thus, the impact of early parenthood on the adolescent processes of separation and individuation is shaped by (a) where in the adolescent process parenthood occurs, (b) how well prepared the adolescent was, prior to parenthood, to engage these tasks of adolescence, and (c) the capacity of the adolescent's family to provide a nurturant environment that is sensitive to the developmental needs of both the adolescent mother and her child.

Ego Identity

Ego identity development in adolescence focuses on tasks inherent to the internalization of an adult personality structure (Erikson, 1958; Josselson, 1987; Cote & Levine, 1987). The processes of ego identity formation in adolescence require a reorientation of interpersonal relationships (e.g., the relationship between child and parent), an expanded view of possible roles for the self and the consolidation of emerging ego strengths.

Ego identity refers to specific characteristics of personality structure which are construed as either ego strengths or deficits and which are manifested in (a) drive organization,

(b) the capacity for impulse control, (c) cognitive complexity, (d) quality of defensive structures, and (e) the capacity for relationship and work commitments. Ego identity refers not only to "who one is" but also to "how one feels about one's self," and to "what one does" (Josselson, 1987).

Erikson (1958) viewed identity development as a life-long process. However, because of the depth and breadth of the cognitive, social, psychological, and physical changes occurring during adolescence, this life phase was deemed the "identity stage" of development in Erikson's model. A primary assumption in Erikson's model of identity development is the idea that separation and individuation are important precursors to identity attainment. More recently, several theorists have suggested that the focus on individuation as a precursor to the capacity for intimacy may be more descriptive of the traditional male experience in our society and that it devalues the traditionally female characteristics of affiliation and cooperativeness (Kroger, 2000). Other empirical investigations of identity development in adolescence have begun to go beyond the traditional components of identity to reflect the importance of domains such as relational experience and commitments, which are constructs clearly relevant to our understanding of parenthood (Grotevant & Cooper, 1986).

As with the processes of separation and individuation, when parenthood occurs during adolescence, the processes of ego identity development may be disrupted (Quinn, Newfield, & Protinsky, 1985). Although adolescents are able to become parents without engaging in emotionally intimate relationships, the tasks of parenting require a consistently high level of intimate engagement. And although the normative tasks of identity development during adolescence often include the "trying on and taking off" of various social roles, the successful adaptation to motherhood requires a strong commitment to a particular social role (Mercer, 1986). Thus, it is important to understand not only how the adolescent's level of identity development affects current parenting capacity, but also how the tasks of parenthood may influence ongoing identity development and thus, future parenting capacity.

Few studies have explored the ways in which ego development during adolescence may affect parenting capacity. And yet, the psychological correlates of identity attainment are important predictors of parenting competence. These include the internal regulation of self-esteem, an internal locus of control orientation, and consistent differentiation of self and other. Among adult mothers, higher levels of identity development are associated with maternal sensitivity Thus, adolescent mothers require support to maintain their own developmental progress toward identity achievement while coping with the potentially contradictory demands of early parenthood.

Cognitive Development

Many of the gains associated with cognitive development during adolescence are relevant to aspects of parenting capacity. The attainment of formal operational thought expands the individuals' capacity to think abstractly, to self-reflect, and to consider the impact of current behavior on future outcomes. The related capacities to see one's self as others might, to see one's own role in relationship to particular situations, and to accurately conceptualize one's relationships to other people each permit the adolescent a greater degree of insight and more accurate judgment.

Another hallmark of cognitive development during adolescence is the emergence, and then diminution, of "adolescent egocentrism" (Elkind, 1974). Early and middle adolescents are often characterized as "egocentric," believing that other people are as focused on their ideas and appearance as they are themselves. Elkind (1967) refers to this phenomenon as the *imaginary audience*. Over time, as adolescents invest more psychological energy into other relationships and external foci, the imaginary audience lessens and the adolescent is better able to relate to others as separate individuals with needs and concerns of their own.

Adolescents who become mothers while still maintaining a high level of egocentrism may be unable to accurately perceive and/or respond to a child's intentions or needs. A baby may continue to be seen as more of a reflection of the adolescent mother's own needs than as a separate person with reality-based needs of her own. For example, an adolescent mother who sees her 3-month-old crying may say, "She's just mad because we're still at school." This statement, although a misperception of an infant's cry signal, may be derived from the young adolescent's inability to take the perspective of the child.

All parents do some "learning how to parent" by trial and error, learning from mistakes and abstracting from such experiences in ways that remediate their future actions (Whitman et al., 1987). Adolescent mothers may be limited by being more bound to concrete operational thinking and thus, may have a more difficult time abstracting from present to future experiences. The idea that adolescent mothers may be more concrete in how they conceptualize parenting also has implications for the development of interventions. Many parent education programs are designed to "teach" about child developmental milestones. Interventions designed for adolescents must be primarily present focused and concrete in nature.

In summary, the cognitive immaturity of adolescent mothers may contribute to deficits in parenting competence. Adolescent egocentrism and concrete operational thinking may interfere with the development of empathic parenting behavior. These normative developmental indices of adolescence may contribute to adolescent maternal behavior that is sometimes found to be less empathic, less contingently responsive, and less appropriate than the behavior of adult mothers.

Stages of Adolescent Development and Implications for Parenting Capacity

It has become standard practice to divide adolescence into three subphases: early, middle, and late (Anthony, 1979; Blos, 1967). Each subphase is marked by particular developmental challenges and milestones of progressive development.

Each stage of adolescence is temporally bounded by normative age ranges. However, because the rate of development varies both within and across individuals, these chronological boundaries may be only loosely correlated with developmental achievement and capacity (Freud, 1965; Hatcher, 1976). The construct of *developmental age* is utilized to denote the extent of an individual's achievement vis-à-vis the tasks of this life phase.

Early Adolescence

The onset of puberty is an important marker of entry into adolescence as well as an event that presents a series of developmental challenges. Adolescents at this stage must simultaneously accommodate increases in hormonal and drive activity as well as begin to integrate a new body image derived from the emergence of secondary sexual characteristics. Early adolescents are often beginning to make preliminary efforts toward a renegotiation of dependence and autonomy with regard to their families of origin. Each of these processes, adaptation to an evolving body image and movements toward autonomy, may be met with ambivalence by adolescents at this stage. Hatcher (1976) observed that this ambivalence may be "seen" in mismatched sets of behavior such as the proclamation of "separateness" from one's own mother while also finding a "best friend" in another adult female role model such as a teacher.

Psychodynamic models of adolescent development often describe the early adolescent's need to divest energy from parental figures, in an effort to support the processes of separation and individuation, and invest this energy into peer relationships (Blos, 1967). Thus, the peer culture surrounding the adolescent during pregnancy and parenthood is likely to be important (Dacey & Travers, 2002). Similarly, the typical defenses of adolescents at this age combine with other factors, such as the fragility of a newly forming body image, to shape the experience of pregnancy and parenthood in particular ways (Hatcher, 1976; Schamess, 1991).

The physical changes associated with puberty may make it difficult for a girl in early adolescence to identify signs of pregnancy. The often heard claim of "not knowing" about a pregnancy becomes more understandable when put in the context of the changing body characteristics associated with puberty such as an increase in body fat, weight gain, irregular menarche, and growth spurts. When a girl in early adolescence is able to acknowledge the reality of a pregnancy, other developmental characteristics may impede her ability to respond adaptively. Early adolescents often have limited cognitive flexibility and limited capacity for abstraction and future orientation. These characteristics may limit the extent to which she is able to perceive the needs of a developing pregnancy or, after birth, a developing child with needs that are separate from her own. For example, it is not uncommon to hear a young adolescent say, "I'm not hungry, so I'm not going to eat today," ignoring the developing child's nutritional needs.

Hatcher (1976) found that, during pregnancy, early adolescents were not able to draw realistic pictures about how their baby would look as an infant. The stick figures drawn by younger adolescents did not have individualized characteristics, and the adolescents never drew themselves performing maternal functions such as holding, feeding, or playing. Among adult mothers, the process of identification with the developing child as well as with the maternal role usually begins during pregnancy (Mercer, 1986). From a cognitive perspective, the adolescent mothers' relative inability to imagine themselves in the future, and/or to abstract the experience of motherhood absent the concrete "trial and error" of having a baby to care for may reflect a normative stage of cognitive development.

Middle Adolescence

The primary developmental challenges faced by middle adolescents reflect their continuing progress toward separation and individuation. Unlike the early adolescent's investment of energy into relationships with peers, the middle adolescent also invests a lot of energy into the self, partially accounting for the narcissism and egocentrism typical of this stage (Elkind, 1974). This shift is supported by the emergence of cognitive capacities at this stage of development that increase the adolescent's ability to be self-reflective and self-aware (Elkind, 1974).

As the middle adolescent becomes less dependent on parental figures and moves toward a state of increased autonomy or interdependence (Hill, 1987), parents are relied on less and less as sources of self-esteem. The adolescent must begin to look inward for self-esteem and affective modulation, relinquishing over time the need for absolute parental approval. The middle adolescent's relationships are often characterized as "moody" because the adolescent engages in, and withdraws from, relationships during this stage (Hatcher, 1976).

Like the early adolescent, middle adolescents continue to be ambivalent about issues relating to autonomy and dependence. Middle adolescents may simultaneously desire autonomy *and* demand that parents "be there" for them. This ambivalence represents real gains in autonomous functioning as well as an increasingly realistic assessment of the difficulties inherent in being on one's own. This state of affairs may create particular conflict with regard to parenthood, because motherhood at this developmental stage often involves a renewed state of dependence on the adolescent's own caregivers.

Adolescents who are in the normative processes of separation and individuation, in early or middle adolescence, or adolescents whose developmental histories make these challenges more difficult present their caregivers with many challenges during the transition to parenthood. As summarized by Schamess (1991), these include (a) Will you continue to love me even if I disappoint you?; (b) Will you prove your love by taking care of me and my child even though I am almost grown up?; (c) What sacrifices are you willing to make for me?; and (d) Will you make those sacrifices willingly and lovingly? (p. 258). The answers of caregivers to these questions may be important determinants of whether the experience of early parenthood will be adaptively incorporated into the adolescent's ongoing development or will more permanently interrupt her developmental progress and capacity for parenthood across time.

Hatcher (1976) found that middle adolescents often viewed their pregnancies as "victories" in relationship to their own mothers. Schaeffer and Pine (1972) describe middle adolescent fantasies of being " a better mother." Statements such as, "I knew my mother would hate me, but I wanted to do it anyway," or "For sure, my mother can't stop me now" are not uncommon. Unlike early adolescents, however, middle adolescents may benefit from many gains in ego strength formulated at this stage. The normative increase in the capacity for abstract thinking allows the middle adolescent to be (a) more self-aware, (b) more realistic, and (c) more future oriented. Thus, the middle adolescent can more realistically consider the consequences of present actions on the future. In addition, as separation–individuation from parental figures continues, the middle adolescent may gain an increased capacity for the internal regulation of self-esteem. Each of these abilities is associated with more sensitive, responsible, and consistent parenting behavior.

Late Adolescence

The primary developmental task of late adolescence is the consolidation of ego identity. Having completed the primary work of separation and individuation, the late adolescent is more capable of sustaining interdependence and reciprocity in relationships. These gains have important

implications for the late adolescent's experience of pregnancy and parenthood.

The late adolescents come closer, than do younger adolescents, to having a "motherly ego" (Deutsch, 1945). Having
resolved primary dependency conflicts, the late adolescent
is more capable of genuine love for others, in addition to the
"self-love" of younger adolescents (Fraiberg, 1980). When
Hatcher (1976) asked late adolescents to draw pictures of
their babies, they were more likely to draw realistic human
figures with individualized characteristics, as well as maternal figures performing nurturant tasks.

Cognitive growth enables the late adolescent to engage
in more effective perspective taking and to more accurately
predict the consequences of their own actions. Each of these
skills is a necessary precursor to empathic parenting (Winnicott, 1965; Beckwith, 1990). As ego identity consolidates,
the capacities for reality testing and the delay of gratification
increase as well. Thus, the late adolescent brings far more
internal resources to the complex tasks of parenthood.

The Social Ecology of Adolescent Parenthood

The processes by which maternal social support affects
child development are varied and complex (Sameroff &
Fiese, 1990). Social support may influence child development indirectly via its effect on parental well-being, attitudes, and parenting behavior, and directly via its effect
on the child's access to other supportive adults such as
friends and relatives (Crnic, Greenberg, Ragozin, Robinson, & Basham, 1983). Studies on adult parents show that
social support buffers against maternal stress are positively
associated with satisfaction in parenting (Crnic et al., 1983),
and correlate positively with self-concept and a belief in
the ability to control one's environment (Veroff, 1981). The
availability of social support is positively associated with
maternal behavior that is more sensitive and involved,
which are characteristics associated with a range of positive child outcomes (Crnic et al., 1983). The presence of
maternal stress, in conjunction with the absence of social
support, is associated with maternal behavior that is more
punitive, negative, and more likely to result in acts of child
abuse and/or neglect (Colleta, 1983).

Adolescent mothers differ from adult mothers not only in their needs for social support, but also in the quality of their social support network and in their capacity to utilize various sources of social support (Kissman & Shapiro, 1990). These differences are best understood in a developmental context that identifies barriers to the adolescent mother's ability to seek out and utilize various sources and kinds of social support.

Among adolescent mothers, the relationship between social support and parenting competence is complex (Shapiro & Mangelsdorf, 1994). "Too much" social support may interfere with the adolescent's maternal role identification and the opportunity for important trial and error learning experiences, compromising her ability to develop parenting skills (Mercer, 1986). For example, if the adolescent's own mother "takes over" the parenting role in an effort to facilitate the adolescent's capacity to finish school, the adolescent is afforded an important developmental opportunity but may need further encouragement to remain involved with the care of her child. This is important because research on the life course of adolescent mothers suggests that it is those adolescents who are able to become independent from their family of origin and create stable relationships who are functioning, as individuals and as parents, most optimally 5 years postpartum (Brooks-Gunn, 1990).

A Note on Interventions and Programs for Adolescent Mothers and Their Children

Over the last several decades, the increasing awareness of the risks associated with adolescent parenthood have led to the development of primary, secondary, and tertiary interventions designed to mediate the effects of early childbearing on the children of adolescent mothers. These programs vary greatly with regard to their primary goals and objectives (Hayes, 1987). The most common objectives include: (a) minimizing obstetrical and neonatal and perinatal complications for both the adolescent mother and her child(ren), (b) fostering parenting skills and optimal parent–child interactions, (c) reducing the social isolation of the adolescent mother, her infant, and her family, (d) promoting economic independence via educational and training opportunities, (e) preventing early repeat pregnancies, (f) supporting the social, emotional, physical, and cognitive development of children born to adolescent mothers, and (g) attending to the ongoing development needs of the adolescent mother herself (Hayes, 1987). As would be expected from the developmental paradigm described in this chapter, these programs almost always have a dual perspective. Specifically, most of these programs are premised on the idea that supporting the development of the adolescent mother is an important component of supporting the developmental well-being of her child(ren).

As is true of all work with children and adolescents, it is necessary that programs for this population focus both on current needs and interventions designed to support the long-term developmental competence of both adolescent mothers and their children. Because there is such wide heterogeneity in the population of adolescent mothers and their children, it is important that particular mother–child dyads receive the kinds of intervention that are matched both to their particular set of needs and capacities to utilize various interventions.

Several practice concerns are important to consider in designing primary, secondary, and tertiary care programs for adolescent mothers and their children. These include (a) defining "who the client is," (b) differentiating among levels of risk, (c) the need for interventions focused on the "here and now," and (d) the need for multigenerational solutions that focus not only on the mother–child dyad, but also on the fathers of children born to adolescents and the extended families of the adolescent mother. Each of these is considered briefly below.

Defining Who the Client Is

Working with adolescent mothers and their children is sometimes complicated by confusion regarding the definition of who the client is. Depending on the specific goals of a program, the primary client may be the adolescent mother, her child(ren), or the relationship between them. For example, programs focused on encouraging high school completion may define their primary "client" as the adolescent mother. However, in order to support the adolescent's ability to stay in school, other program components focused on the adolescent's child (e.g., child care) may also be important. Similarly, programs focused on the physical health and development of children born to adolescent mothers may focus primarily on the provision of care to the adolescent's child. However, these programs may find that unless the needs of the adolescent mother are being addressed, it may be difficult to engage in a prevention program on behalf of her child.

Defining who the client is is also important to the process of program evaluation. Program designers and evaluators need to specify the structure and content of particular programs and the ways in which a given program is expected to alter the life course and/or developmental outcomes of either the adolescent mother or her child(ren). It is important that synchrony exists between the goals of a particular program and the conceptualization of the target population.

Differentiating Levels of Risk

The study of adolescent parenthood raises questions not only regarding normative development during adolescence, but also regarding the occurrence of "off-timed" or unexpected life events, as well as issues presented by subcultural and individual cohort variation. In addition, to fully explore the range of adaptation observed within the population of adolescent mothers and their children, it is necessary to understand normative and nonnormative development in adolescence (Schamess, 1991). Thus, rather than being a unified population at a homogenous level of "risk," adolescent mothers and their children are heterogeneous, characterized by multiple patterns of risk and resiliency with regard to a range of important developmental outcomes. For example, very young adolescents may face different challenges with regard to parenting than adolescents who are older. Likewise, adolescents at equivalent points of psychological maturation may become parents in environments that differ dramatically with regard to other factors associated with parenting competence, such as socioeconomic status. And lastly, adolescents who come to parenting with a history of developmental competence are likely to experience the adaptation to parenthood differently than adolescents whose developmental history is characterized by a range of developmental problems or delays (Schamess, 1990).

Developmental Considerations

The developmental tasks of adolescence are important to consider in designing intervention programs for adolescent mothers. Many indices of developmental maturity are relevant to the adolescent's need for and capacity to utilize a range of intervention strategies. For example, the cognitive maturity of the adolescent is important to consider. Adolescents are more likely, by nature, to be focused on the present and have more difficulty in abstracting from current experiences to future outcomes and behavior. Thus, it is important that programs for adolescent mothers provide ample hands-on and trial-and-error learning opportunities. In addition, the relative cognitive immaturity of adolescent mothers may hamper their capacity to engage in processes such as problem solving. Because many interventions involve problem solving components, it is important to consider how the concrete and/or egocentric nature of adolescent thinking might impact the adolescent's ability to utilize such intervention components.

The Need for Multigenerational and Ecologically Valid Solutions

As research has highlighted, adolescent parenthood presents challenges not only for adolescent mothers and their children, but also for their extended families. To increase the ecological validity of programs for adolescent mothers, it is important to consider the ways in which early childbearing exerts influence on adolescent's' parents and extended family and on fathers of children born to adolescent mothers. Often, the adolescent's own mother may take on a primary caregiving role with regard to the adolescent's child(ren). Although an important source of social support and protection to the development of the child, this shared caregiving may create conflict in the relationship between the adolescent mother and her own parent(s). Such conflict might be anticipated given the normatively adolescent wish to be increasingly autonomous from, and less reliant on, her own parents and family of origin. Solutions to this dilemma require a multigenerational focus that addresses the sometimes conflicting needs and stresses of the adolescent mother, her family of origin, and her child(ren). Similarly, programs designed for adolescent mothers would do well to take into account the nature of the adolescent's relationship with the father of her child. Although fathers of children born to adolescent mothers may not themselves be adolescents, it is worthwhile to try to understand the nature of the relationship between the adolescent mother and the father of her child, as well as the relationship between the adolescent father and the developing child.

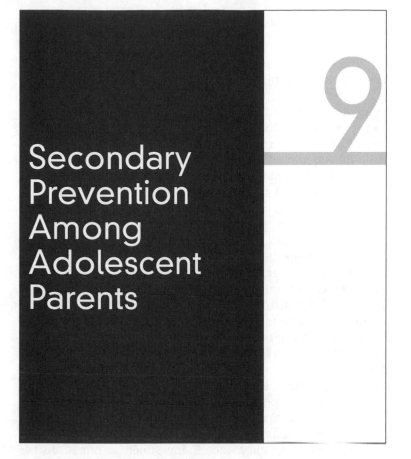

Secondary Prevention Among Adolescent Parents

9

The preponderance of our society's resources directed toward reducing pregnancy and childbearing among adolescents is focused on primary prevention; that is, encouraging young women and men who do not have children to delay their first pregnancy beyond adolescence. Although in recent years subsequent births to teen parents have declined as have first births, they continue to represent a significant proportion of teen births (Widmayer, Adler, & deCubas, 2005), Among all births to adolescents each year, a little over 20% are to teens who already have at least one child (Klerman, 2004). Of these births to teen mothers, about 17% are second births, and 3% are third and higher order births. This means that approximately one-quarter of teen mothers have another child before they turn 20.

There is ample evidence that teenagers who bear one child are at greater risk than other teens for a variety of problematic outcomes across their lifespan. The evidence convincingly suggests also that children of teen mothers disproportionately experience difficulties in a range of indicators of well-being from infancy onward to adulthood. Having additional children during adolescence, especially if the births are closely spaced, conventionally defined as within 18 months to 2 years, increases these risks for both mothers and their offspring. Teen mothers who have more than one child tend to attain lower levels of education, thus lower levels of economic well-being and self-sufficiency. Teen mothers during subsequent pregnancies are more likely to delay seeking prenatal care, have higher risk for preterm delivery, have a baby of low or very low birth weight, and face a greater chance of infant mortality (Kerman, 2004). Children of teen mothers who have another child tend to attain lower levels of education and are more likely to exhibit behavioral problems. The consequences of a rapid additional birth for children likely result from the challenge of providing adequate attention to another young child in context of their struggles as a young and disadvantaged parent. Despite important evidence by Furstenberg (2007) and others of individual differences and heterogeneous outcomes among teen parents and children of teen parents, there is need to redress the imbalance in investment of our resources to work more vigorously to help prevent teen parents from having subsequent children too quickly.

Previous chapters proposed a continuum of risk for adolescents engaging in sexual behaviors that make them vulnerable to pregnancy and contracting sexually transmitted infections (STIs). Despite the fact that the potential of primary prevention programs to successfully reduce teens' likelihood of these outcomes is modest, interventions that are fairly narrowly focused on changing teens' intentions and/or their capacities to act on those intentions do decrease many teens' risky sexual behaviors. Although not all teen mothers share equal likelihood of having more children before reaching adulthood, their overall level of risk of pregnancy is no longer potential: they are, by definition, high-risk youth who face multiple and significant challenges to moving into adulthood well-prepared to fulfill their individual potential for independence and success. Adding to the seriousness of their own difficulties are the consequences to their children of giving birth again within a short time.

This does not mean that the life trajectory of a teen mother, or her child, is determined the moment she gives birth. On the contrary, many teenage parents and their children proceed through life facing primarily the predictably unpredictable problems in living that all families experience. Like all families, they carry forward the legacy of past generations' emotional and relational patterns, and bear the exigencies of historical context and of their unique individuality. However, other families begun by teenagers also experience particular difficulties associated with the typical developmental features of the parents' youth as explicated in the previous chapter. It is hard to overcome this dual set of demands in achieving healthy individual and family development when teenagers already have one child. However, young parents who have a second or third child are more likely to be disadvantaged in ways that make it even harder to overcome the inherent stresses of youthful parenthood. Effective secondary prevention for teen parents extends far beyond providing requisite knowledge and skills to reduce episodes of unprotected sex and thus the risk of pregnancy. Secondary prevention for teen parents must provide comprehensive support for their own psychosocial development as they adapt to the early transition to the many adult roles that accompany parenthood as well as support for the health and well-being of their children.

In placing findings of three decades following the original group of teen mothers and their children from his seminal study in Baltimore in context, Furstenberg (2007) observes:

The problems that researchers face in assessing the causal effect of early childbearing arise from the fact that teenager childbearing does not occur randomly. Early parenthood happens disproportionately to adolescents (and their partners) who are different in a variety of ways from the teens who typically delay parenthood. Think of it this way: who is more likely to become pregnant and bring the pregnancy to term—a girl who has limited cognitive abilities, has failed a grade or two, and is attending a very poor high school where early parenthood is common, or a girl who is a strong student, gets considerable praise from her teachers, and is in a program for college-bound students. The answer is obvious, but this difference in the proclivity of certain teenagers to have children—to "select themselves" into the role—creates enormous headaches for researchers who want to identify whether and how much teenage childbearing causes later outcomes. How much is the effect of early childbearing due to the preexisting differences between early and later childbearers, and how much is due to the timing of the first birth?...Another way of characterizing the findings of the Baltimore study—as well as the results of the more methodologically sophisticated research—is that teenage childbearing is more a consequence than a cause of economic and social disadvantage. (pp. 7, 51)

This conclusion leads Furstenberg to argue that rather than focusing on adolescent pregnancy prevention per se, the wiser strategy to improve youth well-being is to reduce poverty and social disadvantage and hence eliminate the most powerful and entrenched sources of risk. The validity of his analysis is supported by the concentration of early childbearing among the most disadvantaged young women and men; and especially teen parents who have additional children without changing the essential individual and environmental conditions into which their first child is born. Without engaging here the important larger implications of Furstenberg's argument about macro level, social and economic change, suffice it to acknowledge that this perspective highlights the immense difficulty in reducing high-risk sexual behavior—the immediate behavioral cause of teen pregnancy—in the face of deeply complex forces at work among youth who may see few alternatives in their future and compromised means for creating such alternatives. This is why primary prevention among the highest risk teenagers is difficult, and why secondary prevention among teen parents is even more difficult. This difficulty is exacerbated by a tendency among researchers, policy architects, and service providers alike to avoid engaging fully the profoundly complicated psychological and sociocultural dimensions of teen parents' life circumstances and histories. Instead, much research focuses on examining relationships among variables without plumbing the phenomenological meaning and multidimensional nature of the constructs; while programs for teen parents and their children often do not attend adequately to the deeply psychological as well as social dimensions of the clients' typically impoverished and highly stressed lives. Greater success in helping teen parents avoid the most worrisome outcomes will require deepening and expanding how we understand and respond to these vulnerable young families. That said, there is sufficient knowledge to provide some insight into the circumstances of teen parents, guide risk–assessment, and intervention priorities, if not well-developed practice guidelines.

Subsequent Births: Risk Factors

Despite an uncomfortable—and slightly acknowledged—element of happenstance in which sexually active teenage girls conceive or boys impregnate them, there are identifiable and predictable degrees and kinds of risk of unprotected sexual activity that can result in an unplanned pregnancy. Unlike the voluminous literature that identifies clearly the multiple antecedent factors associated with high-risk sexual behaviors and their consequences among nonparenting adolescents, the knowledge base regarding teen parents is more limited and more ambiguous. The problem of a relative dearth of reliable information about subsequent births to teens is compounded by the overarching problem of establishing the direction of causality articulated above.

While it is likely that many of the same forces at play among nonparenting teens influence the sexual behavior of teen parents, we know far less about which ones are more or less important in each decision along the path to subsequent pregnancies. In addition, these individual factors exist in a substantively different context when a young person has a child and is coping with the multiple, complex, and sometimes conflicting demands of adolescence and parenthood. Below we review ways in which teen mothers who have subsequent births are distinct relative to other teen mothers, with the objective of identifying implications for effective secondary prevention services.

Age of Teen Mother

Most studies find that the older the teen is at first birth, the more likely she is to have a second child (Klerman, 2004). However, there are inconsistent findings based both on varying samples and methods of data analysis, suggesting that younger teens are more likely to have a second child and within a shorter time. Until there is more reliable evidence to clarify this question, the findings of Manlove et al. (2000) provide adequate working assumptions. In a frequently cited study based on a large and nationally representative sample of teen mothers, they found that, "...a disturbingly high proportion of the youngest teen mothers eventually had a second birth, a pattern due primarily to a longer risk period for these teens. After controlling for background characteristics, however, younger and older teens showed a similarly high risk of subsequent births..." (p. 443). This implies that age alone is less important than the types of individual, family and other environmental circumstances in which a teen mother has her first child.

Race/Ethnicity of Teen Mother

The race or ethnicity of a teen mother is more clearly associated than age with her propensity to have an additional child. Poor white mothers are slightly more likely than non-poor white mothers to have a closely spaced birth. Rates of additional and especially closely spaced births are higher among black and Hispanic teen mothers than among white teen mothers in general (Klerman, 2004). Yet we do not know to what degree and the means by which racial and ethnic identity influences young parents' sexual and parenting behavior. Some literature posits that cultural norms and expectations within some low-income black communities and families favor teen parents having additional children quickly, but there is insufficient evidence to evaluate directly the plausibility of this view.

Marital Status/Relationship with the Baby's Father

Although marriage among teen parents occurs infrequently today, when the teen mother is married at the time of the first birth and remains married, or marries the baby's father within 2 years, she is more likely to have another child as a teenager. More common than marriage, however, is cohabitation of a teen mother and her boyfriend. Some studies find that between one third and one half of young fathers live with their child's mother at the time of the birth (Cutrona et al., 1998; Carlson, 2004). Other research suggests that over one third of children of teen fathers see them every day (Stouthamer-Loeber, M. and Wei, 1998; Fagot, et al, 1998).

Living with her boyfriend—or another adult who is not her parent—increases a teen mother's chance of having a closely spaced subsequent birth. When the baby's father helps provide childcare the couple is also more likely to have another child. In general, then, the more regular contact the adolescent parents have, the more likely they are to conceive again. This may be so because of the potential for increased sexual contact or because the teen mother feels that the baby's father has a commitment to their family, thus is more inclined to have another child with him.

This relationship presents complex issues that currently are not well understood (Cutrona, Hessling, Bacon, & Russell, 1998). Generally, the presence of a child's father is considered desirable, and there is increasing effort to encourage young fathers to be more involved in their children's lives. At the same time, closer connection between the teen mother and her partner increases the chances of a closely spaced second or third birth. Interventions should attend to helping couples consider the consequences of having more children soon after the first. The difficulty in achieving this is made more complicated as teen fathers can bring their own sources of risk to the relationship, including low academic performance and early school dropout (Xie, Cairns & Cairns, 2001; Stouthamer-Loeber & Wei, 1998, low family income (Fagot et al., 1998; Xie, Carins & Cairns, 2001), antisocial behavior (Fagot et al, 1998), high arrest rates (Thornberry, Smith, & Howard, 1997), deviant peer association (Fagot et al., 1998; Xie, Cairns, & Cairns, 2001) and living in neighborhoods characterized by poverty (Thornberry, Smith, and Howard, 1997). Of course, not all young fathers have all, or even any, of these characteristics that are associated with fathering a teen birth. However, assessing risk of subsequent births to an adolescent mother must include the father's own set of circumstances as a potentially potent source of influence on fertility outcomes and the future well-being of the young parents and their children.

In addition, as Musick (1993) so powerfully argues, teen mothers whose own early childhood was fraught with poverty, family chaos, and dysfunction often struggle with emotional and psychological issues related to unmet needs for love, affiliation, and nurturing. These unresolved issues may result in a desire to have an additional child with their baby's father as a way to increase his commitment to her. The importance of this lens on teen parents' motivation for change will be addressed further in regard to prevention strategies.

Living Arrangements

In contrast to the impact of living with her boyfriend, teen mothers who live with one or both of their parents are less likely to have another child within 2 years (Klerman, 2004). Parents who provide assistance in caring for a teen's child can enable her to be more engaged in school, thus increasing her ability to complete more education, which is strongly connected to delaying a subsequent pregnancy (Manlove, et al., 2000). However, there is inconsistent evidence about whether the protective impact of the family can be compromised when grandparents take on the role of primary caretaker in place of the young mother. Interestingly, teen mothers who live on their own with their child are also less likely to have to have another child, for reasons that have not been well studied (Manlove, et al., 2000).

There is little research that examines directly how a teenage parent's family environment might influence subsequent childbearing. However, based on her study of the relationship between teen pregnancy and parenting on families, Corcoran (2001) concludes that secondary prevention programs should "address the parenting teen's family functioning, particularly in the areas of problem-solving, communication, roles, and behavior control" (p. 47). Despite the implied concerns about the quality of familial dynamics, the evidence clearly shows the potential benefits to teen mothers' educational trajectory when they reside with parents who are able to support her efforts to remain in school. These findings are especially important given the requirements that teen parents live with parents or adult guardians in order to qualify to receive Temporary Assistance for Needy Families (TANF) benefits.

Educational Achievement and Attainment and Cognitive Ability

The role of educational achievement and attainment in long-term well-being highlights the difficulty of disentangling "cause" and "effect" in subsequent childbearing among teen parents. Teens who drop out of school before becoming pregnant are more likely to have a closely spaced subsequent birth, as are teen mothers who drop out after giving birth and do not return. In contrast, teens who remain in school after the birth of their child and go on to obtain a high school diploma or GED are more likely to delay a second birth.

These observations, reflecting widespread consensus among practitioners and scholars, reasonably suggest that being in school, an age-appropriate activity for an adolescent, helps protect young women from multiple early births. However, the decision to drop out or to remain in school is, as Furstenberg asserts, not random, nor is it independent of a variety of other important influences on the adolescent's educational trajectory. Some of these influences derive from being a teen parent; while others exist, or preexist, in her school or community environment and interact with her individual attributes. For example, teens who attend schools with more economically disadvantaged students are more likely to have an additional birth, regardless of their individual educational performance (Manlove, et al., 2000). This points to the potential impact of peer norms and attitudes that support, or at least do not negatively sanction teen motherhood.

There is also growing evidence that teen mothers who have lower cognitive ability are significantly more likely to have another child quickly, perhaps as much as three times as likely as teen mothers with higher cognitive ability (Klerman, 2004). Teen mothers who have lower education expectations for themselves also are more likely to have additional children soon. The potential meaning of intellectual aptitude is evident in research showing that teen mothers who were in classes or programs for gifted children also tend to delay subsequent pregnancy. However, it is not clear to what extent the advantages conferred by the enriched educational environment can be separated clearly from the advantages of greater cognitive capacity. In addition to naturally possessing greater reasoning and problem-solving skills that protect them, it may be that young people who excelled early in school benefited from a better education and were encouraged to see themselves as capable and promising. They may also have been surrounded by peers who had higher expectations for their futures, thus expect more for themselves. These questions require further in-depth study in order to tease out the direction of various factors associated with education and teenage childbearing. In any event, it is unambiguously clear that teen parents who remain engaged in their education are at lower risk for another birth as a teen, and are making a critically important investment in their future self-sufficiency and ability to care for their children.

Desire to Have an Additional Child

Perhaps one of the least studied, hence least understood, yet potentially important influences on teen parents having another child within a short time is whether they intended to have the first child and, how they feel about having a second child. There is a growing body of evaluation studies of secondary prevention programs that concludes that some teen mothers (the typical client population of prevention programs) do not benefit from the intervention because, "Finally, in some communities, rapid second births among adolescent mothers may be valued and regarded as desirable, thereby undermining many intervention programs" (Black et al., 2006).

There is little well-conceptualized literature directly exploring the assumption that a primary motivation for subsequent teen births is the positive value place on having more than one child closely spaced. There are a few studies that directly inquire about the intentions of teen mothers to become pregnant soon after they deliver or their reactions to becoming pregnant again. Yet, this research does not shed much light on the motivation for further childbearing, especially because there tends to be surprisingly low correlation between teen mothers' predictions of when and if they will conceive again and their actual fertility outcomes.

A few studies comparing teen mothers who have additional children with those who delay childbearing interpret findings of, for example, higher self-esteem among those with a second infant as indirect evidence that they desired the child (Black, et al., 2006). To an extent, then, the attribution of intention is an inference based on limited ability to explain such behaviors as the failure of some teen mothers to use contraception consistently, or their propensity not to make risk-reducing choices about education, employment, or relationships with men. Beyond the list of individual-level factors listed above that constitute a profile of relative risk and, on one hand, the speculation about the impact of community norms and values that encourage early childbearing on the other, there does not yet exist a coherent and theoretically based literature accounting for why some teen mothers might "want" more children quickly, and what that desire means to them.

One important exception to the largely a-theoretical approach both to explaining and intervening in subsequent childbearing among particularly disadvantaged teen mothers is the work of Judith Musick, whose ecologically contextualized emphasis on adolescent development draws on many years of working with teen mothers at the Ounce of Prevention Fund in Chicago. In considering the costs as well as rewards that inhere in having another baby, Musick observes:

> *Is a subsequent pregnancy a sign of program failure? Sometimes it is, but not always. More important, it is a marker and reminder that for disadvantaged girls fertility is often the arena in which change is played out. For a teenage mother, decisions about having another child are often psychological moments of truth, intimately connected to her will and ability to redirect her life, to decide then stick to the decision to live in a new way. The risks are those of separation from people she cares about and of going from the known to the unknown—without assurances that she will be able to make it in a vast, less familiar world. It may also call for her to be secure enough to deny fatherhood to a new partner, at least for the present. (1993, p. 212)*

In other words, what appears "simply" as a positive desire for additional children soon after a teen gives birth, may, in fact, reflect deep emotional and psychological responses to the young person's choices for her future. What to a social science researcher or program staff member is clearly a risk to her and her baby's future may, to the young mother, offer the opportunity to meet other, more compelling immediate needs. With that observation, let us now turn to what we know does—and does not—help a young mother make such important judgments about risk.

Secondary Prevention Programs. The recently mounting evidence regarding effective approaches to helping teen parents circumvent the risks attending early parenthood provides one clear and strong conclusion: prevention is difficult to achieve. The evidence leads to this conclusion, primarily because teen parents generally face complicated and numerous problems that require multifaceted and intensive forms of assistance over time. In addition, it is difficult to find clear evidence-based direction for practice because the great variety of programs for teen parents is not easily compared. The problem of generalizing from the promising but varying findings of effectiveness is compounded by methodological limitations posed by many weakly designed evaluations.

Diverse programs for teen parents and pregnant teens, loosely categorized as "prevention," differ greatly in their objectives hence their services. Program objectives range widely and typically include some combination of helping pregnant teens and teen parents deliver healthy infants, return to and remain in school, obtain vocational training, increase financial independence, use contraception, be better parents, and delay having another child past adolescence (Black, et al., 2006; Coren, et al., 2003; East, et al., 2003; Klerman, 2004; Philiber, et al., 2003; Sangalang, et al., 2006; Sangalang, 2006; Sims & Luster, 2002; Sangalang & Rounds, 2005; Solomon & Solomon, 2008; Stevens-Simon, 2000). Some programs also provide services directly to young children of teen parents. Thus, although "secondary prevention" implies the prevention of a teen parent having another child, programs vary in how directly they approach the goal, implicitly expanding the purview of prevention to include other aspects of well-being. In other words, the very definition of "prevention" among pregnant and parenting teens and their children is conceptually and practically complex. Nevertheless, despite the somewhat inchoate state of the field and the knowledge upon which practice is based, the evaluation of literature provides some important lessons. In a similar process to Kirby's (2007) review of the most rigorous program evaluations available, Klerman (2004) synthesized descriptive findings about major dimensions of program structure and function and their impact on service outcomes. Based on her analysis of rigorously evaluated programs, let us review the landscape of program elements and then focus on how they affect the quality of services, especially success in delaying subsequent births.

Service Location and Type

Service location and type vary widely, including multisite, multiservice community-based programs, school-based services, alternative schools, medical clinics, and home-visiting, none of which independently appear to confer a clear advantage on outcomes. In South Carolina, the Second Chance Club provides services to urban high school students in school, a university medical clinic, and in their homes. In Elmira, New York and Memphis, Tennessee, a long-running program sends nurses in to the homes of pregnant teens and continues visits through 2 years postpartum. The Polly T. McCabe Center in New Haven, Connecticut offers educational, social, and medical services to pregnant teens and then selected services after they deliver. Among these various types of programs, there is no clear advantage to any of them. Rather, the most important feature of more effective programs appears to be *"the strength of the relationship built between the teenage mother and the individual working with her"* (Klerman, 2004, p. 26).

Program Personnel

Program personnel have diverse backgrounds and levels of professional training and expertise. Whether personnel are providing services through home visiting or in a formal agency setting, programs whose staff are professionals rather than paraprofessionals or lay people tend to have greater positive impact in client outcomes. Although it is common to use staff effectively whose background are closer to those of their clients in order to enhance the ability to "relate" to their circumstances and experiences, act as role models, and enhance community legitimacy, Musick and Stott (2000) note some potential limitations in their capacities to serve disadvantaged mothers. They observe that often paraprofessionals, "lack easy access to mainstream institutions and organizations that are vital pathways to success" (p. 200). They are also "more likely to be hampered by their own inadequately resolved problems around sexuality, relationships to men, childrearing practices, family violence, assertiveness, or autonomy" (p. 200). If part of professional training includes autonomy based on specialized knowledge and skills, and for mental health professionals, a strong self-awareness to enhance the conscious use of self, it stands to reason that lay staff may be more prone to identify too closely with their clients. Musick and Stott suggest more specifically three possible limitations to effective service. First, they draw on Halpern's notion of "domains of silence" to describe those areas of painful emotional vulnerability based on unresolved past experiences that can prevent a worker from openly addressing certain issues with a client. Second is the risk of unexamined countertransference that can have "powerful psychological reverberations for service providers because they are so heavily affect-laden and may threaten to bring into awareness feelings so painful they have been denied or repressed" (p. 447). Finally, community para-professionals may transfer low expectations they had of their own children to their clients, thus not pushing them to achieve their highest potential. Musick and Stott suggest that such low expectations may derive from a sense of powerlessness or helplessness based on their own "internalizations of poverty and discrimination" (p. 447). They go on to suggest how good supervision, clear role expectations and training can help mitigate some these risks. Nevertheless, it is important to consider carefully what characteristics are most important in serving teen parents whose needs may require high levels of expertise to address well.

Service Initiation and Length

Service initiation and length appear to be important, but not in systematically verified patterns. Some programs begin services when teens are pregnant, others after they deliver or even later. The current body of research findings about effectiveness does not provide enough information to know the independent significance of whether services are initiated pre- or postpartum.

There is more compelling evidence regarding the significance of length of involvement in a program. More successful programs of diverse types, such as the comprehensive community program, Parents Too Soon, and the Elmira and Memphis visiting home nurse programs, involve teen parents for at least 2 years postpartum. Several programs that had only short-term success in delaying births attribute their very modest outcomes to termination of services by the agency or poor retention of clients. We do not know exactly what about length of service receipt accounts for greater success, but obvious possibilities include the impact of a sustained relationship with staff over the course of facing new demands in childrearing and adolescent development into young adulthood.

Major Emphasis

Major emphasis among programs varies widely. Klerman (2004) observes, "Although all the programs reviewed included preventing additional pregnancies and births among their goals, it appeared that many were more concerned with healthy pregnancies and infants, return to school, and high school graduation" (p. 27). Among the programs included in Klerman's review, the programmatic emphasis did not have any discernible impact on how well they helped teen parents delay additional pregnancies or births. Rather the impact of successful program appears to derive from other elements, especially in the presence of strong relationships between the young people and program personnel.

Attention to Family Planning

Attention to family planning would seem to be a self-evidently important emphasis in effective pregnancy prevention. However, in light of the disparate methods of delivering family planning services and the resulting difficulty in comparing outcomes, no firm conclusions are possible. The unsurprising notable exception to this lack of clear evidence is that programs that facilitate teen mothers receiving contraceptive implants show strong effects in the length of time to subsequent pregnancy. In addition, nurses tend to be more skilled than staff of other backgrounds in providing effective contraceptive counseling and referral.

Practice Implications

Despite the rather limited empirical basis for designing specific methods of effective secondary prevention strategies for teen parents, we are able to identify some principles that can form the foundation of various types of programs. As with any good program planning, of course, the first task is to define the target client population and their needs, as was discussed in previous chapters. Not all pregnant and parenting teens are, by virtue of their community, background, and individual characteristics, necessarily extremely disadvantaged. However, by virtue of their circumstances as young parents they are highly likely to have needs with such a wide span that a comprehensive emphasis is necessary to have a real and a lasting impact on them and their children. Based on the assumption of broad needs that continue over time, several general practice guidelines follow.

1. **The program should encourage and facilitate pregnant and parenting teens' educational attainment and achievement**. Enhancing educational engagement means lowering barriers to returning to and remaining in school as well as supporting teens' motivation and capacities as students. This may be achieved in an alternative school setting or programs within the school that are flexible and responsive to the particular demands of being a parent. This may also be achieved in programs not situated in schools through collaboration with educational institutions on behalf of pregnant and parenting teens. The daily struggle of a teen parent to organize herself and her child can itself be overwhelming and overtax her internal and external resources. Thus, concrete services like childcare and transportation, academic support and career guidance, as well as emotional sustainment, may all be necessary for a teen parent to cope with the simultaneous demands of being a parent and student. In addition, students who have low cognitive ability and those who have not had prior educational success need special attention in order to continue their education and delay subsequent births.

2. **The program should provide the knowledge, skills and means necessary to prevent unwanted pregnancy.** We know that emphasizing family planning alone is not effective, and that we do not know precisely the best method of providing family planning services to teen parents. Nevertheless, as a matter of sheer logic and practicality, it is also clear that teens who are sufficiently motivated to want to prevent pregnancy must have the capacity to do so. These services may be provided by qualified program staff or through referral to the appropriate provider. Family planning counseling is best conducted in an individual rather than group setting. It should include providing reliable and specific information about all types of birth control, their benefits and drawbacks, help in learning how to use a chosen method correctly, and support to try different methods if so desired. Teen mothers should be encouraged to use long-lasting and non-coital–dependent methods such as hormone injections or the patch. In addition, teen

parents should have easy access to contraception, including emergency contraception. Providing teen parents with knowledge, resources, and support will not alone create the intention to avoid pregnancy; but it may increase their competence and confidence, thereby reinforcing the belief that they can determine whether they conceive or have another child. Teen parents often use contraception faithfully for the first 6 months postpartum, but decrease their vigilance to prevent another pregnancy thereafter. This suggests that family planning services should be designed to take into account the developmental stage of the teen as a parent as well as her age. When this service occurs one-on-one with a professional staff person, it is also possible to explore in greater depth the strongly influential non-sexual issues surrounding contraception such as the relationship with her (or his) romantic partner and the meaning of becoming pregnant.

3. **Program personnel must be professionally trained. Nonprofessional staff should receive close supervision by appropriate professional staff.** Depending upon the type of services provided to pregnant and parenting teen, the staff who are delivering the services should have the appropriate professional background to respond to their clients' complex multiple needs with a high level of skill and authority. Paraprofessionals and other lay people can provide various meaningful and competent services, for example, as peer mentors or community visitors, but they should receive extensive training and ongoing supervision.

4. **The program should provide each pregnant and parenting teen the opportunity to develop a close, sustained, and reliable relationship with an adult.** This is perhaps the most important element of each successful program, regardless of the program's emphasis, location, or methods of intervention. A close relationship can provide or enhance existing motivation for a young parent to carry out the difficult work to overcoming ongoing and emerging challenges and meet long-term goals. This requires that aspects of the services delivered are based on individual, face-to-face contact rather than through groups, and at least some times in the teen's home. This good working relationship must be sustained over time, preferably 2 years postpartum.

5. **Services should engage the teen's family when feasible.** Although many teen parents' families of origin are themselves sources of some of the risks they carry into young parenthood, teens should be encouraged to live with their families or guardians if they be helped to provide economic, social, and/or emotional support (Klerman, 2004). The client system should be conceptualized broadly beyond the teen, and perhaps her child, to include those individuals who are potential sources of support and who exert influence on the young parent. In reflecting on how families can exacerbate the crises that may accompany transitions necessary to improve a young parent's life circumstances, Musick (1993) observes, nonetheless, that, "Well-considered interventions can circumvent such crises by helping girls resolve issues that cannot be worked out in their families. They should not encourage or actively help the girls move out of their homes unless it is absolutely necessary" (p. 219).

Summary

Just as all good practice is predicated on addressing the particular reality of each individual, so practice with teen parents must begin where they are. Meeting teen parents there requires the commitment and the capacity to engage them far more meaningfully, more deeply, with more sophisticated knowledge and skills than often is present in secondary prevention programs. Such practice is costly, not only in material resources but those characterizing a potentially intense, long-term relationship that can provide a supplement to flagging energy, motivation, and vision to a young parent whose opportunities to thrive may be thwarted by the demands of young parenthood. The potential ultimate cost of not meeting those needs, however, is too high for them and for the larger society to bear.

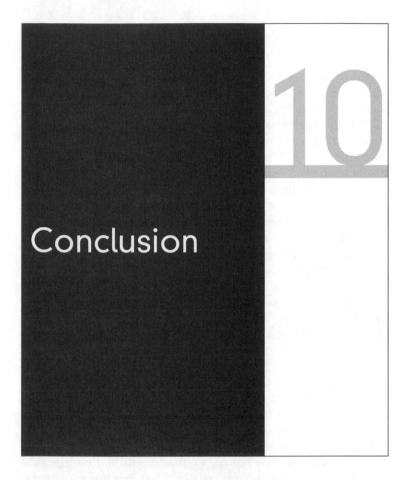

Conclusion

At an annual meeting of Adolescent Family Life program grantees a few years ago, a presenter asked participants, mainly program administrators and professional researchers, how many had ever had sex, not wishing to become pregnant, without using birth control. Naturally, nearly everyone in the room raised their hands. The question, of course, was intended to illustrate that most of us, regardless of background or intelligence, are capable of acting on impulse in ways that might bring unintended consequences such as pregnancy. The shock of self-recognition was powerful, the point well taken.

Despite the obvious truth of this observation about human nature, there is something misleading about it in the larger context of adolescent pregnancy today. Although most people of all ages make serious mistakes in judgment on occasion, not all people—not all young people—are equally likely to become single teenage parents. Despite the continuing widespread incidence of sexually transmitted infections (STIs) among teenagers, the contrast between those young people who navigate adolescence avoiding pregnancy and parenthood and those who become young parents is, in some respects, increasing.

The preceding chapters have documented extensively the contours of such differential risk. Having argued at length that such differences do exist, the following few facts about a young woman whom I met recently emphasize *why* it is important to distinguish carefully among the various meanings of early, unprotected sex and pregnancy.

At age 20, Billie is unmarried and the mother of a 5-year-old boy, being raised by her own mother, and a 5-month-old girl. Although she has almost "lost" her children to the Department of Social Services more than once, Billie believes that they are the reason she is able to "go on" living and keep her dream of becoming a nurse. She must travel a long road to reach that goal. Billie, having completed only 9th grade, has been in jail several times for drug-related offenses, and is desperately poor. She became pregnant when she was 14 years old, soon after becoming sexually active. Like distressingly numerous other young women, she says she deliberately had sex with a boy so that her own father would not be "the first one." Her father had been sexually molesting her for several years, and she was determined that he not be the man to finally "take" her virginity. Choosing her first sexual partner at age 14 seemed to be a way for Billie to assert some control over a life filled otherwise with emotional and physical violation, poverty, family chaos, and distress. Birth control was far from her consciousness.

In the scheme of Billie's short and traumatic life, having become a teenage mother may not have been the single most influential event in her subsequent experiences. Early, unprotected sex and pregnancy may also not be conceptual "keys" to understand Billie's behavior patterns over her life thus far. They are, nevertheless, deeply comprehensible, however regrettable, facts in the overall course of her development. She did not simply make an error in judgment or give in to the heat of the moment. It is probable that no sex education class—assuming she had stayed in school—would have prevented her from becoming a young mother. The significance of this point is heightened when we consider that although

Billie, like most other mothers, is absolutely sincere in her love and desire to make a better future for her children, they were born in to profoundly worrisome circumstances.

Billie and her children are not unusual in their plight. Although they are a numeric minority among our society's families, their needs are disproportionately intense and urgent. Thus, distinctions in the meanings of and motivations for young people's sexual behavior as suggested here repeatedly have importance well beyond meeting the formal requirements of sound research and theory. Our capacity to provide meaningful services that help young people compensate for vulnerabilities, build on capacities, and develop to healthy adulthood rests on making accurate distinctions among youths' needs and circumstances and responding accordingly through a wide range of coordinated efforts. Several implications for practice and research follow from this perspective.

One implication is the need to nurture an increasing collective willingness to conceptualize teen pregnancy prevention as a community-wide concern and responsibility. This growing willingness is evident in the numerous state-level initiatives that provide different kinds of supports to local communities. Some states provide primarily information or an "umbrella" administrative structure to constituent organizations. Others provide financial and technical resources directly to organizations or local governmental units. Regardless of variety in expression, deliberately intensifying public awareness and commitment to prevention is essential to maintaining current positive trends in pregnancy and STI reduction among adolescents. The significant decline in rates of childbearing among American adolescents in recent decades suggests that concerted attention to reducing their sexual risk-taking can have a real impact on their behavior. At the same time, the current rise in those rates is worrisome, and also highlights the need for vigilance in maintaining the high level of public awareness as today's young children approach adolescence, facing the same risks as their older siblings and neighbors did.

To the degree that there is explicit public "ownership" of prevention efforts, members of communities will openly discuss difficult questions such as the relative responsibilities of public and private spheres for providing sexuality education and how to best invest public resources for youth and family development that are consistent with their values, traditions, resources, and other local characteristics. Open debate and consideration of these difficult matters are necessary to overcome the inevitable conflicts arising from differences in political, ideological, religious, cultural, and other affiliations that can stymie change. In spite of genuine value conflicts among members of communities, it is both possible and crucial to continue encouraging the kind of social conservatism that gives young people pause for thought before becoming sexually active or having sex without protection. In addition to being an essential condition for developing effective policies and services, open acknowledgement of the many issues connected with teenage sexuality and risks of pregnancy and STIs communicates to young people that adults are aware of their developmental challenges and are willing to provide them with guidance as they face difficult choices.

Necessary as this condition of public ownership is, it is not sufficient for meeting the needs of all youths. Another important development is the growing interest in defining teenage pregnancy prevention and services as aspects of enhancing youth development rather than as singular solutions to a narrowly understood problem. Although optimal development, seen as the capacity to meet the various demands of adult functioning, is the overall goal of youth services, pregnancy prevention does not mean simply trying to regulate sexual activity. Rather, it means helping individual young women and men actively envision and concretely move toward a future that might be endangered by short-sighted choices such as unprotected intercourse. In its broadest application, this orientation suggests that social workers should routinely consider reducing the risks of early sex and pregnancy to be an integral aspect of services across problem areas, levels of practice, and practice contexts rather than only specialized settings.

At the same time, this orientation also directs our attention to the specific needs of the most at-risk young people, for whom the possibility of early childbearing is both more likely and more devastating than for others. Those youths who are more distant from creating positive visions of their future and even farther from having the capacity to reach them require more formal, targeted intervention by social workers and others who promote social welfare. Aggressive efforts to prevent school drop out, address mental health problems and drug and alcohol use, and enhance educational and occupational potential and opportunity are aspects of pregnancy prevention in the most meaningful sense for vulnerable children and youths. These young people ought disproportionately to occupy our professional attention in general, especially if we wish to reduce early childbearing outside of marriage.

Consistent with a perspective on teenage pregnancy-related services that is based on youth development and differential risk, research should continue to examine with greater nuance what approaches "work" best with which young people in reducing unprotected sexual activity. A continuing glaring gap in our knowledge is how ethnic and other cultural differences among young people affect their patterns of sexuality and which prevention approaches are most helpful. Research reports too often treat the issue of generalizability in a routine way, with little in-depth analysis of what factors might affect how young people of differing characteristics respond to a program. This tendency accounts for some of the difficulty in reaching reliable conclusions overall about the effectiveness of program approaches and their components.

This problem is compounded by the great variety in programs, their constituent intervention activities, and the fact that they may implicitly be targeting dissimilar antecedent factors and using widely varying outcome measures. These problems can be mitigated somewhat by deliberately identifying target antecedents and then matching them more closely with program elements; that is, using the principles of a logic model outlined in chapter 6. Although these problems are being addressed incrementally by the steadily accumulating body of literature that results from more stringent requirements for evaluation by most sources of support for services, there is much room for improvement in the quality of design of most studies of programs.

Of course, underlying the technical methodological difficulties is the fact that, in the end, pregnancy prevention services cannot easily assess their substantive raison d'etre, which is delaying pregnancy and childbearing until adulthood. By definition, this requires longitudinal methods, a difficult research requirement for most program evaluations to fulfill. In better studies, the objectives evaluated mirror the program objectives. These often include behaviors—such as increased knowledge, changed intentions, and so on—that are proximate outcomes believed to mediate longer-term pregnancy outcomes. Assuming the theories are correct about what factors influence adolescents' sexual behavior, expectations of evaluation research center can reasonably emphasize methodological rigor and transparency. However, although many more program evaluations use behavioral outcomes such as pregnancy or childbirth, many studies of teen pregnancy-related programs still use process outcomes, a relatively weak type of information. Although we need not belabor the inherent challenges of agency-based research, this limitation seriously hampers our ability to identify how and why programs affect clients' behavior.

Despite the limitations in the current evaluation literature on teenage pregnancy prevention services, we actually know a great deal about what inhibits and what facilitates child and adolescent development, including the dynamics of sexual activity. The cumulative knowledge base of social work, drawing as it does on multiple disciplines and research traditions, provides a strong foundation from which to craft good services. The dynamic and heterogeneous nature of our society affects the substance and the context of our service in innumerable and shifting ways; yet, we have fundamental wisdom about timeless human needs such as nurturance through meaningful relationships, a valued place in the larger community and society, and the opportunity to develop individual potential. When these basic needs are more or less satisfied, young people need relatively minimal intervention, focusing primarily on imparting developmentally appropriate knowledge and skills in order to delay childbearing until adulthood. However, if such needs are inadequately satisfied, more comprehensive and intensive intervention—especially a close relationship with a caring adult—is indicated to avoid unprotected sex and other co-occurring problem behaviors. It certainly is not possible to prevent all teenagers from becoming pregnant or contracting an STI. We can, however, continue our current progress in reducing the overall incidence of unplanned and early pregnancy among young people. It is also possible, and of most pressing importance, to reduce the troubling and intergenerational consequences of childbearing among our nation's most vulnerable youths through aggressive efforts at prevention. At this juncture, our more serious barrier to achieving these objectives is finding the professional and public will to act on what we already know that will lead youths to well-functioning and productive adulthood.

Appendix A

State Laws on Minors' Access to Abortion

State	Minors' Access	Public Funding	State Legislation 2008
Alabama	Requires written consent of at least one parent except in cases of medical emergency, abuse, assault, incest, or neglect. Judicial bypass is available for mature minor.	No public funding is available unless abortion is necessary to preserve the life of the woman or pregnancy results from rape or incest.	
Alaska	Consent only. Enforcement is permanently enjoined by court order; policy not in effect.	Public funding is available for all or for most medically necessary abortions with court order.	
Arizona	Requires written consent of one parent except in cases of medical emergency. Judicial bypass is available for mature minor.	Public funding is available for all or for most medically necessary abortions with court order.	

(continued)

State Laws on Minors' Access to Abortion (continued)

State	Minors' Access	Public Funding	State Legislation 2008
Arkansas	Requires written consent of at least one parent except in cases of medical emergency, abuse, assault, incest, or neglect. Judicial bypass is available for mature minors who are able to give informed consent or if in best interest of minor. State-directed abortion counseling and a wait until the following day required.	No public funding is available unless abortion is necessary to preserve the life of the woman or pregnancy results from rape or incest.	
California	Consent only. Enforcement is permanently enjoined by court order; policy not in effect.	Public funding is available for all or for most medically necessary abortions with court order.	
Colorado	Requires notification of at least one parent in person or by certified mail at least 48 hours before except in cases of medical emergency or in cases of abuse, assault, incest, or neglect. Judicial bypass is available if minor is sufficiently mature or if in best interest of minor.	No public funding is available unless abortion is necessary to preserve the life of the woman or pregnancy results from rape or incest.	

State	Minors' Access	Public Funding	State Legislation 2008
Connecticut	Minor, age 12 and older, may consent to abortion services (no parental involvement required). Abortion counseling is required to obtain informed consent.	Public funding is available for all or for most medically necessary abortions with court order.	
Delaware	Requires notification of at least one parent for minors who are younger than the age of 16, exceptions are made in cases of medical emergency or if another adult relative agrees parental consent not in minor's best interest. Judicial bypass is available for mature minors.	No public funding is available unless abortion is necessary to preserve the life of the woman or pregnancy results from rape or incest.	
District of Columbia	Minor, age 12 and older, may consent to abortion services (no parental involvement required).	No public funding is available unless abortion is necessary to preserve the life of the woman or pregnancy results from rape or incest.	

(continued)

State Laws on Minors' Access to Abortion (continued)

State	Minors' Access	Public Funding	State Legislation 2008
Florida	Requires notification of at least one parent except in the case of a medical emergency. Judicial bypass is available for mature minor.	No public funding is available unless abortion is necessary to preserve the life of the woman or pregnancy results from incest or rape.	
Georgia	Requires notification of at least one parent except in the case of a medical emergency. Judicial bypass is available for mature minor.	No public funding is available unless abortion is necessary to preserve the life of the woman or pregnancy results from incest or rape.	
Hawaii	No restrictions as of 2008.	Public funding is available for all or for most medically necessary abortions with court order.	
Idaho	Requires written consent of at least one parent except in cases of medical emergency, abuse, assault, incest, or neglect. Judicial bypass is available for mature minor.	No public funding is available unless abortion is necessary to preserve the life of the woman or pregnancy results from incest or rape.	State law prohibits coercing a woman into having an abortion.

State	Minors' Access	Public Funding	State Legislation 2008
Illinois	Notification only. Enforcement is permanently enjoined by court order; policy not in effect.	Public funding is available for all or for most medically necessary abortions with court order.	
Indiana	Requires written consent of at least one parent except in cases of medical emergency, abuse, assault, incest, or neglect. Judicial bypass is available for mature minor.	No public funding is available unless abortion is necessary to preserve the life of the woman or pregnancy results from incest or rape. Other exceptions include physical health.	
Iowa	Requires notification of at least one parent in person or by certified mail 48 hours before, except in cases of medical emergency, abuse, assault, incest, or neglect. Other adult relatives may be involved in lieu of parent. Judicial bypass is available if minor is mature and capable of informed consent or if in best interest of minor.	No public funding is available unless abortion is necessary to preserve the life of the woman, there are fetal abnormalities, or the pregnancy is a result of rape or incest.	

(continued)

State Laws on Minors' Access to Abortion (continued)

State	Minors' Access	Public Funding	State Legislation 2008
Kansas	Requires notification of at least one parent except in cases of medical emergency, abuse, neglect, assault, or incest. Judicial bypass is available if minor is mature and well informed or if in best interest of minor.	No public funding is available unless abortion is necessary to preserve the life of the woman, or the pregnancy is a result of rape or incest.	
Kentucky	Requires written consent of at least one parent except in cases of medical emergency. Judicial bypass is available for mature minor.	No public funding is available unless abortion is necessary to preserve the life of the woman, or the pregnancy is a result of rape or incest.	
Louisiana	Requires consent of at least one parent except in cases of medical emergency. Judicial bypass is available.	No public funding is available unless abortion is necessary to preserve the life of the woman, or the pregnancy is a result of rape or incest.	

State	Minors' Access	Public Funding	State Legislation 2008
Maine	Minors, age 12 and older, can consent to abortion services (no parental involvement required) according to Guttmacher. Written consent of at least one parent and minor (if younger than 18 yrs old) is required. Judicial bypass is available for mature minor or if in best interest of minor. Abortion counseling is required for informed consent.	No public funding is available unless abortion is necessary to preserve the life of the woman, or the pregnancy is a result of rape or incest.	
Maryland	No restrictions as of 2008.	Voluntarily funds all or most medically necessary abortions.	
Massachusetts	Requires written consent of one parent except in cases of medical emergency. Judicial bypass is available for mature minor.	Public funding is available for all or for most medically necessary abortions with court order.	

(continued)

State Laws on Minors' Access to Abortion (continued)

State	Minors' Access	Public Funding	State Legislation 2008
Michigan	Requires written consent of one parent except in cases of medical emergency. Judicial bypass is available for mature minor.	No public funding is available unless abortion is necessary to preserve the life of the woman, or the pregnancy is a result of rape or incest.	
Minnesota	Requires notification of both parents 48 hours before except in cases of medical emergency, abuse, assault, incest, or neglect. Judicial bypass is available.	Public funding is available for all or for most medically necessary abortions with court order.	
Mississippi	Requires consent of both parents except in cases of medical emergency. Judicial bypass is available.	No public funding is available unless abortion is necessary to preserve the life of the woman, there are fetal abnormalities, or the pregnancy is a result of rape or incest.	

State	Minors' Access	Public Funding	State Legislation 2008
Missouri	Requires informed written consent of at least one parent. Judicial bypass is available for well-informed minor with mental and intellectual capacity to consent or if in best interest of minor.	No public funding is available unless abortion is necessary to preserve the life of the woman or the pregnancy is a result of rape or incest.	
Montana	Requires notification of at least one parent. Enforcement of this law is permanently enjoined by the court.	Public funding is available for all or for most medically necessary abortions with court order.	
Nebraska	Requires written notification of at least one parent except in cases of medical emergency, abuse, neglect, assault, or incest. Judicial bypass is available for mature minor.	No public funding is available unless abortion is necessary to preserve the life of the woman or the pregnancy is a result of rape or incest.	

(continued)

State Laws on Minors' Access to Abortion (continued)

State	Minors' Access	Public Funding	State Legislation 2008
Nevada	Requires personal notification of at least one parent. Notification is not necessary in cases of medical emergency. Enforcement of this law is permanently enjoined by the court. Abortion counseling is required.	No public funding is available unless abortion is necessary to preserve the life of the woman or the pregnancy is a result of rape or incest.	
New Hampshire	No restrictions as of 2008.	No public funding is available unless abortion is necessary to preserve the life of the woman or the pregnancy is a result of rape or incest.	
New Jersey	Requires written notification of at least one parent and 48-hour waiting period, except in cases of medical emergency. Enforcement of this law is permanently enjoined by the court.	Public funding is available for all or for most medically necessary abortions with court order.	

State	Minors' Access	Public Funding	State Legislation 2008
New Mexico	Requires consent of at least one parent. Enforcement of this policy is permanently enjoined by the court.	Public funding is available for all or for most medically necessary abortions with court order.	
New York	No restrictions as of 2008.	Voluntarily funds all or most medically necessary abortions.	
North Carolina	Requires consent of at least one parent except in cases of medical emergency or if other adult relative agrees consent not in minor's best interest. Judicial bypass is available if minor is mature and well informed enough to consent, in cases of rape or incest or if in best interest of minor.	No public funding is available unless abortion is necessary to preserve the life of the woman or the pregnancy is a result of rape or incest.	
North Dakota	Requires consent of both parents except in cases of medical emergency. Judicial bypass is available.	No public funding is available unless abortion is necessary to preserve the life of the woman or the pregnancy is a result of rape or incest.	

(continued)

State Laws on Minors' Access to Abortion (continued)

State	Minors' Access	Public Funding	State Legislation 2008
Ohio	Requires consent of at least one parent. Judicial bypass is available.	No public funding is available unless abortion is necessary to preserve the life of the woman or the pregnancy is a result of rape or incest.	State law requires provider to offer woman options to view image if ultrasound is performed before abortion.
Oklahoma	Requires notification and consent of at least one parent except in cases or medical emergency. Judicial bypass is available.	No public funding is available unless abortion is necessary to preserve the life of the woman or the pregnancy is a result or rape or incest.	State law requires ultrasound, a verbal description of the image, and provider to offer woman to view the image before the abortion. Requires ultrasound equipment in clinics. Allows medical providers and institutions to refuse to provide abortion services.
Oregon	No restrictions as of 2008.	Public funding is available for all or for most medically necessary abortions with court order.	

State	Minors' Access	Public Funding	State Legislation 2008
Pennsylvania	Requires consent of at least one parent except in cases of medical emergency. Judicial bypass is available.	No public funding is available unless abortion is necessary to preserve the life of the woman or the pregnancy is the result of rape or incest.	
Rhode Island	Requires consent of at least one parent. Judicial bypass is available.	No public funding is available unless abortion is necessary to preserve the life of the woman or the pregnancy is the result of rape or incest.	
South Carolina	Minors, younger than age 17, require consent of at least one parent except in cases of medical emergency, abuse, as-sault, incest, or neglect. Other adult relative may be involved in lieu of parent. Judicial bypass is available.	No public funding is available unless abortion is necessary to preserve the life of the woman or the pregnancy is the result of rape or incest.	State law requires provider to offer woman options to view image if ultrasound is performed before abortion.

(continued)

State Laws on Minors' Access to Abortion (continued)

State	Minors' Access	Public Funding	State Legislation 2008
South Dakota	Requires notification of at least one parent except in cases of medical emergency. Judicial bypass is available.	No public funding is available unless abortion is necessary to preserve the life of the woman.	State law requires provider to offer to perform ultrasound before abortion.
Tennessee	Requires consent of at least one parent and documentation of relationship of parent to minor, except in cases of medical emergency, abuse, assault, incest, or neglect. Judicial bypass is available for sufficiently mature, well-informed minors or if in best interest of minor.	No public funding is available unless abortion is necessary to preserve the life of the woman or the pregnancy is the result of rape or incest.	
Texas	Requires signed consent of at least one parent except in cases of medical emergency. Judicial bypass is available if involving parent would put minor at risk of physical or emotional abuse or for mature minors.	No public funding is available unless abortion is necessary to preserve the life of the woman or the pregnancy is the result of rape or incest.	

State	Minors' Access	Public Funding	State Legislation 2008
Utah	Requires notification and consent of at least one parent except in cases of medical emergency, abuse, assault, incest, or neglect. Judicial bypass is available. (The provisions only apply to parental consent requirement.)	No public funding is available unless abortion is necessary to preserve the life of the woman, there are fetal abnormalities, the pregnancy is the result of rape or incest, or there is a threat to the woman's physical health.	
Vermont	No restrictions as of 2008.	Public funding is available for all or for most medically necessary abortions with court order.	
Virginia	Requires consent of at least one parent or other adult relative, except in cases of medical emergency, abuse, assault, incest, or neglect. Judicial bypass is available.	No public funding is available unless abortion is necessary to preserve the life of the woman, there are fetal abnormalities, or the pregnancy is a result of rape or incest.	
Washington	No restrictions as of 2008.	Voluntarily funds all or most medically necessary abortions.	

(continued)

State Laws on Minors' Access to Abortion (continued)

State	Minors' Access	Public Funding	State Legislation 2008
West Virginia	Requires notification of at least one parent except in cases of medical emergency. Judicial bypass is available. Specific health professionals may waive parental involvement if judge is unavailable.	Public funding is available for all or most medically necessary abortions with court order.	
Wisconsin	Requires consent of at least one parent or other adult relative except in cases of medical emergency, assault, abuse, incest, or neglect. Judicial bypass is available. Specific health professionals may waive parental involvement if judge is unavailable.	No public funding is available unless abortion is necessary to preserve the life of the woman, there is a threat to the woman's physical health, or the pregnancy is a result of rape or incest.	State law requires information on emergency contraception for rape victim. Requires emergency contraception provision to rape victim on request.

State	Minors' Access	Public Funding	State Legislation 2008
Wyoming	Requires written consent of at least one parent except in cases of medical emergency. Judicial bypass is available if minor is mature and well informed or if in best interest of minor.	No public funding is available unless abortion is necessary to preserve the life of the woman or the pregnancy is a result of rape or incest.	

APPENDIX B

State Policies for Sexuality and STI/HIV Education

State	Sexuality Education	STI/HIV Education
Alabama	Not mandated Abstinence stressed Contraception covered	Mandated Abstinence stressed Contraception covered
Alaska	Not mandated	Not mandated
Arizona	Not mandated Abstinence stressed (Parental consent required)	Not mandated Abstinence stressed
Arkansas	Not mandated Abstinence stressed	Not mandated Abstinence stressed
California	Not mandated Abstinence covered Contraception covered	Mandated Abstinence covered Contraception covered
Colorado	Not mandated Abstinence stressed Contraception covered	Not mandated Abstinence stressed
Connecticut	Not mandated Abstinence covered	Mandated
Delaware	Mandated Abstinence covered Contraception covered	Mandated Abstinence covered Contraception covered
District of Columbia	Mandated Contraception covered	Mandated
Florida	Mandated Abstinence covered	Mandated

(continued)

State Policies for Sexuality and STI/HIV Education (continued)

State	Sexuality Education	STI/HIV Education
Georgia	Mandated Abstinence covered	Mandated Abstinence covered
Hawaii	Mandated Abstinence stressed Contraception covered	Mandated Abstinence stressed Contraception covered
Idaho	Not mandated	Not mandated
Illinois	Not mandated Abstinence stressed	Not mandated Abstinence stressed Contraception covered (A law requires a school district providing sexuality education to provide statistics on the efficacy of condoms as HIV/STI prevention)
Indiana	Not mandated Abstinence stressed	Mandated Abstinence stressed
Iowa	Mandated	Mandated
Kansas	Mandated	Mandated
Kentucky	Mandated Abstinence covered	Mandated Abstinence covered
Louisiana	Not mandated Abstinence stressed	Not mandated Abstinence stressed
Maine	Mandated Abstinence stressed Contraception covered	Mandated Abstinence stressed Contraception covered
Maryland	Mandated Abstinence covered Contraception covered	Mandated Abstinence covered Contraception covered
Massachusetts	Not mandated	Not mandated
Michigan	Not mandated Abstinence stressed	Mandated Abstinence stressed
Minnesota	Mandated	Mandated Abstinence covered

State	Sexuality Education	STI/HIV Education
Mississippi	Not mandated Abstinence stressed (Localities may override state requirements)	Not mandated Abstinence stressed
Missouri	Not mandated Abstinence stressed	Mandated Abstinence stressed
Montana	Mandated Abstinence covered	Mandated Abstinence covered
Nevada	Mandated (Parental consent required)	Mandated (Parental consent required)
New Hampshire	Not mandated	Mandated Abstinence covered
New Jersey	Mandated	Mandated
New Mexico	Not mandated	Mandated Abstinence stressed Contraception covered
New York	Not mandated	Mandated Abstinence stressed Contraception covered
NorthCarolina	Mandated Abstinence stressed	Mandated Abstinence stressed
Ohio	Not mandated	Mandated Abstinence stressed
Oklahoma	Not mandated Abstinence stressed	Mandated Abstinence covered Contraception covered
Oregon	Mandated Abstinence stressed Contraception covered	Mandated Abstinence stressed Contraception covered
Pennsylvania	Not mandated	Mandated Abstinence stressed
Rhode Island	Mandated Abstinence stressed Contraception covered	Mandated Abstinence stressed Contraception covered
South Carolina	Mandated Abstinence stressed Contraception covered	Mandated Abstinence stressed Contraception covered

(continued)

State Policies for Sexuality and STI/HIV Education (continued)

State	Sexuality Education	STI/HIV Education
South Dakota	Not mandated Abstinence is taught within state-mandated character education	Not mandated
Tennessee	Mandated Abstinence stressed	Mandated Abstinence stressed
Texas	Not mandated Abstinence stressed	Not mandated Abstinence stressed
Utah	Mandated Abstinence stressed (Parental consent required)	Mandated Abstinence stressed (Parental consent required)
Vermont	Mandated Abstinence covered Contraception covered	Mandated Abstinence covered Contraception covered
Virginia	Not mandated Abstinence covered Contraception covered	Not mandated Abstinence covered Contraception covered
Washington	Not mandated Abstinence stressed Contraception covered	Mandated Abstinence stressed Contraception covered
West Virginia	Not mandated Abstinence stressed Contraception covered	Mandated Abstinence stressed Contraception covered
Wisconsin	Not mandated Abstinence stressed	Mandated Abstinence stressed

Source: *The Alan Guttmacher Institute*, 2008.

References

Abadinsky, H. (1997). *Drug abuse: An introduction* (3rd ed.) Chicago: Nelson–Hall, Inc.

Abama, J. C., Martinez, G. M., Mosher, W. D., & Dawson, B. S. (2004). Teenagers in the United States: Sexual activity, contraceptive use, and childbearing. *Vital and Health Statistics, 23*(24).

Afxentiou, D., & Hawley, C. B. (1997). Explaining female teenagers' sexual behavior and outcomes: A bivariate probit analysis with selectivity correction. *Journal of Family and Economic Issues, 18*, 19–106.

Ainsworth, M. D. S., Blehar, M. C., Waters, E., & Wall, S. (1978). *Patterns of attachment.* Hillsdale, NJ: Lawrence Erlbaum Associates.

The Alan Guttmacher Institute (AGI). (1999a). *Teenage pregnancy: Overall trends and state-by-state information.* (April, 1–18). New York: The Alan Guttmacher Institute.

The Alan Guttmacher Institute (AGI). (1999b). *Teen sex and pregnancy. Facts in Brief.* Retrieved July 15, 2000, from http://www.agi-usa.org/pubs/fb_teen_sex.html.

The Alan Guttmacher Institute (AGI). (1999c). *Why is teenage pregnancy declining? The roles of abstinence, sexual activity, and contraceptive use. Occasional Report,* New York: The Alan Guttmacher Institute. Retrieved August 22, 2008, from http://www.agi-usa.org/pubs/or_teen_decline.html.

The Alan Guttmacher Institute (AGI). (2001a). The status of major abortion-related laws and policies in the states. Special Report. Retrieved September 14, 2008, from http://www.agi-usa.org/pubs.abort_law_status.html.

The Alan Guttmacher Institute (AGI). (2001b). *State policies in brief: Parental involvement in minors' abortions.* New York: The Alan Guttmacher Institute.

The Alan Guttmacher Institute (AGI). (2001c). *Minors' access to contraceptive services. State Policies in Brief.* New York: The Alan Guttmacher Institute.

Albarracin, D., Gilletee, J., Earl, A., Glasman, L., Durantini, M., & Ho, M. (2005). A test of major assumptions about behavior change: A comprehensive look at the effects of passive and active HIV-prevention interventions since the beginning of the epidemic. *Psychological Bulletin, 131*(6), 856–897.

Alexander, E., & Hickner, J. (1997). First coitus for adolescents: Understanding why and when. *Journal of the American Board of Family Practice, 10*(2), 96–103.

Allen, J. P., Philliber, S., Herrling, S., & Kuperminc, G. (1997). Preventing teen pregnancy and academic failure: experimental evaluation of a developmentally based approach. *Child Development, 68*(4), 729–742.

Amaro, H., Zuckerman, B., & Cabral, H. (1989). Drug use among adolescent mothers: Profile of risk. *Pediatrics, 84*(1), 144–151.

Anda, R. F., Felitte, V. J., Chapman, D. P., Croft, J. B., Williamson, D. F., Santelli, J., et al. (2001). Abused boys, battered mothers, and male involvement in teen pregnancy. *Pediatrics, 107*, 19–27.

Anderson, S., Gerard, M. S., Dallal, E., & Must, A. (2003). Relative weight and race influence average age at menarche: Results from two nationally representative surveys of US girls studied 25 years apart. *Pediatrics, 111*(4), 844–850.

Anthony, J. (1979). The essential Piaget: An interpretive reference and Guide. *Journal of American Academy of Child and Adolescent Psychiatry, 18*(2), 401–402.

As–Sanie, S., Gantt, A., & Rosenthal, M. (2004). Pregnancy prevention in adolescents. *American Family Physician, 70*(8), 1517–1524.

Babor, T. F., Del Boca, F. K., McLaney, M. A., Jacobi, B., Higgins–Biddle, J., & Hass, W. (1991). Just say Y.E.S.: Matching adolescents to appropriate interventions for alcohol and other drug-related problems. *Alcohol, Health and Research World, 15*(1), 77–86.

Baker, S. A., Thalberg, S. P., & Morrison, D. M. (1988). Parents' behavioral norms as predictors of adolescent sexual activity and contraceptive use. *Educational Psychology, 23*(90), 265–282.

Bandura, A. (1977). *Social learning theory.* Englewood Cliffs, NJ: Prentice Hall.

Barnett, J., & Hurst, C. (2003). Abstinence education for rural youth: An Evaluation of the Life's Walk Program. *Journal of School Health, 73*(7), 264–268.

Barth, R. P., & Schinke, S. P. (1984). Enhancing the social supports of teenage mothers. *Social Casework* (65), 34–43.

Barth, R. P. (1987). Adolescent mothers' beliefs about open adoption. *Social Casework* (June), 323–331.

Bearman, P. S., & Bruckner, H. (1999). *Power in numbers: Peer effects on adolescent girls' sexual debut and pregnancy.* Washington, DC: The National Campaign to Prevent Teen Pregnancy.

Bearman, P. S., Bruckner, H. J., Brown, B. B., Theobald, W., & Philliber, S. (1999). *Peer potential: Making the most of how teens influence each other.* Washington, DC: The National Campaign to Prevent Teen Pregnancy.

Becker, E., Rankin, E., & Rickel, A. U. (1998). *High-risk sexual behavior: Interventions with vulnerable populations.* New York: Plenum Press.

Becker, G., Landes, E.M., & Michael, R. (1977). An economic analysis of marital instability. *Journal of Political Economy, 85*(6), 1141–1185.

Becker, P., (1987). Sensitivity to infant development and behavior: A comparison of adolescent and adult single mothers. *Research Nursing Health,* 10, 119–127.

Becker, R. (2000). Male involvement and adolescent pregnancy prevention. ETR Associates. Retrieved from http://www.etr.org.recapp. theories.mip.index.htm

Beckwith, L. (1990). Adaptive and maladaptive parenting: Implications for intervention. In S. Meisels & J. Shonkoff (Eds.), *Handbook of early childhood intervention.* Cambridge, MA: Cambridge University Press.

Bellis, M. A., Downing, J., & Ashton, J. R. (2006). Adults at 12? Trends in puberty and their public health consequences. *Journal of Epidemiology and Community Health, 60,* 910–911.

Belsky, J. (1984). The determinants of parenting: A process model. *Child Development, 55,* 83–96.

Benda, B. B., & DiBlasio, F. A. (1991). Comparison of four theories of adolescent sexual exploitation. *Deviant Behavior, 12*, 235–257.

Benda, B. B. (2002). The effects of various aspects of religion and family on ad olescent sexual behavior. *Marriage and Family: A Christian Journal, 5*(3), 373–390.

Benedek, T. (1959). Parenthood as a developmental phase: A contribution to libido theory. *Journal of the American Psychoanalytic Association, 7*, 389–417.

Bennett, S., & Assefi, N. (2005). School-based teenage pregnancy preventions: A systematic review of randomized controlled studies. *Journal of Adolescent Health, 36*(1), 72–81.

Benson, P. L., Scales, P. C., Hamilton, S. F., & Sesma, A., Jr. (2006). Positive youth development for far: Core hypotheses and their implications for policy and practice. *Search Institute, 3*(1), 1–13.

Billy, J. O. G., Brewster, K. L., & Grady, W. R. (1994). Contextual effects on the sexual behavior or adolescent women. *Journal of Marriage and the Family, 56*, 387–404.

Black, M. M., Bentley, M. E., Papas, M. A., Oberlander, S., Teit, McNary, L. O, et al. (2006). Delaying second births among adolescent mothers: A randomized controlled trial of a home-based mentoring program. *Pediatrics, 18*(4), 1087–1099.

Blaikie, A. (1995). Motivation and motherhood: Past and present attributions in the reconstruction of illegitimacy. *The Sociological Review,* 640–656.

Blos, P. (1962). *On adolescence: A psychoanalytic interpretation.* New York: The Free Press.

Blos, P. (1967). The second individuation process of adolescence. *The Psychoanalytic Study of the Child, 22*, 162–186. New York: International Universities Press.

Blum, R. W., Beuhring, T., Shrew, M. L., Bearinger, L. H., Sieving, R. E., & Resinck, M. D. (200). The effects of race, income and family structure on adolescent risk behavior. *American Journal of Public Health, 90*(12), 1879–1984.

Blume, S. B. (1992). Alcohol and other drug problems in women. In J. H. Lowinson, P. Ruiz, R. B. Millman & J. G. A. E. Langrod (Eds.), *Substance Abuse: A Comprehensive Textbook* (2 ed., pp. 794–807). Baltimore: Williams & Wilkins.

Blythe, M. J., Fortenberry, J. D., Temkit, M., Tu, W., & Orr, D. (2006). Incidence and correlates of unwanted sex in relationships of middle and late adolescent women. *Archives of Pediatric Medicine, 160*, 591–595.

Boggess, S., & Bradner, C. (2000). Trends in adolescent males' abortion attitudes, 1988–1995: Differences by race and ethnicity. *Family Planning Perspectives, 32*, 118–123.

Boonstra, H. (2000). Welfare law and the drive to reduce "illegitimacy." *The Guttmacher Report on Public Policy.* New York: The Alan Guttmacher Institute.

Borakowski, E., Trapl, M., Lovegreen, L., Colabianchi, N., & Block, T. (2005). Effectiveness of abstinence-only intervention in middle school teens. *American Journal of Health Behavior, 29*(50), 423–434.

Bower, B. (1997). Mental disorders tied to teen parenthood. *Science News, 52*(15), 229.

Bowlby, J. (1969). *Attachment and Loss: Volume 1. Attachment.* New York: Basic Books.

Boyer, C. B., Tschann, J. M., & Schafer M. (1991). Predictors of risk for sexually transmitted diseases in ninth grade urban high school students. *Journal of Adolescent Research, 14*(4), 448–465.

Bragg, E. J. (1997). Pregnant adolescents with addictions. *Journal of Obstetric Gynecologic and Neonatal Nursing, 28*(6), 623–627.

Brewster, K. Cooksey, E., Grulkey, D., & Rindfuss, R. (1998). The changing impact of religion on the sexual and contraceptive behavior of adolescent women in the United States. *Journal of Marriage and the Family, 60*(2), 493–504.

Brewster, K. L. (1994). Neighborhood context and the transition to sexual activity among young black women. *Demography, 31*(4), 603–614.

Brewster, K. L. (1994). Race differences in sexual activity among adolescent women: The role of neighborhood characteristics. *American Sociological Review, 59*, 408–434.

Brewster, K. L., Billy, J. O. G., & Grady, W. R. (1993). Sexual context and adolescent behavior: The impact of community on the transition to sexual activity. *Social Forces, 71*, 713–740.

Briffault, R., & Malinowski, B. (1956). *Marriage past and present.* Boston: Porter Sargent Pub.

Brindis, C. (2006). A public health success: Understanding policy changes related to teen sexual activity and pregnancy. *Annual Review of Public Health, 27*, 277–295.

Brindis, C., & Philiber, S. (2003). Improving services for pregnant and parenting teens. *The Prevention Researcher, 10*(3). Retrieved October 12, 2008, from http://www.tpronline.org.

Brooks-Gunn, J. (1990). Adolescents as daughters and as mothers: A developmental perspective. In I Sigel & G. Brody (Eds.), *Methods of family research: Volume 1.* Hillsdale, NJ: Lawrence Erlbaum Associates.

Brooks-Gunn, J., Duncan, G.J., Klebanov, P.K., & Sealand, N. (1993). Do neighborhoods influence child and adolescent development? *American Journal of Sociology, 99*(2), 353–395.

Brooks–Gunn, J., & Furstsenberg, F. (1986). The children of adolescent mothers: Physical, academic and psychological outcomes. *Developmental Review, 6*, 224–251.

Browning, C. R., & Laumann, E. O. (1997). Sexual contact between children and adults: A life course perspective. *American Sociological Review, 62*, 540–560.

Brown, N.K. (2003). Relapsing, Running, and Relieving: A Model for High Risk Behavior in Recovery. *Journal of Addictions Nursing, 14*(1), 11–17.

Buffardi, A., Thomas, K., Homes, M.D., & Manhand, L. (2008). Moving upstream: Ecological and psychosocial correlates of sexually transmitted infections among young adults in the United States. *American Journal of Public Health, 98*(6), 1128–1136.

Buhi, E. R., & Goodson, P. (2007). Predictors of adolescent sexual behavior and intention: A theory-guided systematic review. *Journal of Adolescent Health, 40*(2007), 4–21.

Burtless, G. (1994). Public spending on the poor: Historical trends and economic limits. In S. H. Danziger, G.D. Sandefur & D.H. Weinberg (Eds), *Confronting poverty: Prescriptions for change*. Cambridge: Harvard University Press.

Burton, L. M. (1990). Teenage childbearing as an alternative life-course strategy in multigenerational black families. *Human Nature, 1*(2), 123–143.

Carlson, M. J. (2004). Involvement by young, unmarried fathers before and after their baby's birth. *The Prevention Researcher, 11*(4). 14–17.

Carlton, R. (2001). South Carolina Department of Health and Environmental Control, *Youth Leadership Initiative*, Office of Youth Development.

Carpenter, S. C., Clyman, R. B., Davidson, A. J., & Steiner, J. F. (2001). The association of foster care or kinship care with sexual behavior and first pregnancy. *Pediatrics, 108*(3), 1–6.

Carrera, M. A. (1995). Preventing adolescent pregnancy: In hot pursuit. *Siecus Report, 23*(6), 16–19.

Carter–Jessop, L., Franklin, L., Heath, J., Jiminez–Irazarry, G., & Peace, M. (2000). Abstinence education for urban youth. *Journal of Community Health, 25*(4), 293–304.

Cassidy, J., & Shaver, P. (Eds.). (1999). *Handbook of attachment: Theory, research and clinical implications*. New York: Guilford Press.

Cassidy, B., Zoccolillo, M., & Hughes, S. (1996). Psychopathology in adolescent mothers and its effects on mother-infant interactions: A pilot study. *Canadian Journal of Psychiatry, 41*, 379–384.

Caudill, H. (1963). *Night comes to the Cumberlands*. Boston: Little, Brown and Co.

Center for Addiction and Substance Abuse (CASA). (1999). *Dangerous liaisons: Substance abuse and sex*. Funded by The Henry J. Kaiser Family Foundation. The Carnegie Corporation of New York: December.

Centers for Disease Control and Prevention. (1997). Alcohol Consumption Among Pregnant and Childbearing-Aged Women—United States, 1991 and 1995. *Morbidity and Mortality Weekly Report. 46*(16), 346–350.

Centers for Disease Control and Prevention. (1998). *Tobacco Use Among U.S. Racial/Ethnic Groups: A Report of the Surgeon General – Executive Summary*. Washington, DC: U.S. Department of Health and Human Services.

Centers for Disease Control and Prevention. (2008). Trends in HIV-and STD-Related risk behaviors among high school students—United States 1991–2007. *MMWR, 57*(30), 817–828.

Center for Law and Social Policy. (2000). *CLASP Update*, February 2000. Available at: http://www.clasp.org/pubs/clasptupdate/Cufeb2000. htm. Retrieved December 8, 2000.

Chase–Lansdale, P. L., & Brooks–Gunn, J. (1995). *Escape from poverty: What makes a difference for children?* Cambridge: Cambridge University Press.

Chase–Lansdale, P. L., Brooks–Gunn, J., & Paikoff, R. (1991). Research and programs for adolescent mothers: Missing links and future promises. *Family Relations, 40*, 396–402.

Child Welfare League of America. (2008). *CWLA 2008 Children's Legislative Agenda*. Retrieved April 8, 2009, from http://www.scla.org/advocacy.2006 legagenda15.htm.

Children's Defense Fund. (1985). *Preventing children having children.* Washington DC: Children's Defense Fund.

Childtrends. (2001). Retrieved November 1, 2001, from http://childtrends.org/

Chilman, C. S. (1979). *Adolescent sexuality in a changing American society: Social and psychological perspectives.* Washington, DC: U.S. Government Printing Office.

Christopher, F. S., Johnson, D. C., & Roosa, M. W. (1993). Family, individual, and social correlates of early Hispanic adolescent sexual expression. *Journal of Sex Research, 30*(1), 54–61.

Christopher, F. S. (1995). Adolescent pregnancy prevention. *Family Relations, 44*, 384–391.

Chumlea, W. C., Schubert, C. M., Roche, A. F., Kulin, H. E., Lee, P. A., Himes, J. H., & et al. (2003). Age at menarche and racial comparisons in U.S. girls. *Pediatrics, 11*(1), 111–113.

Clark, J. (1971). Adolescent obstetrics: Obstetrical and societal roles. *Clinical Obstetrics and Gynecology, 14*(5), 1026–1036.

Clark, K. (1965). *Dark ghetto.* New York: Harper and Row.

Cobliner, W. G. (1974). Pregnancy in the single girl: The role of cognitive functions. *Journal of Youth and Adolescence, 3*(1), 17–28.

Colcord, J. C. (1923). The need of adequate case work with the unmarried mother. *The Family, 4*(7), 167–172.

Coletta, N., & Gregg, C. (1981a). Adolescent mothers' vulnerability to stress. *Journal of Nervous and Mental Disease*, 50–54.

Coletta, N., & Gregg, C. (1981b). How adolescents cope with the problems of early motherhood. *Adolescence, 16*, 499–512.

Colletta, N., & Lee, D. (1983). The impact of support for black adolescent mothers. *Journal of Family Issues, 4*, 127–143.

Cook, C. (1997). The role of the social worker in perinatal substance-abuse. *Social Work in Health Care, 24*(3–4), 65–83.

Corcoran, J. (2000). Multi-systemic influences on the family functioning of teens attending pregnancy prevention programs. *Child and Adolescent Social Work Journal, 18*(1), 37–49.

Cote, J., & Levine, C. (1988). A critical examination of the ego identity status paradigm. *Developmental Review, 8*(2), 147–184.

Cox, J., & Bithoney, W. (1995). Fathers of children born to adolescent mothers: Predictors of contact with their children at 2 years. *Archives of Pediatric and Adolescent Medicine, 149*, 962–966.

Coyle, K., Kirby, D, Parcel, G., Basen–Engquist, K., Bahspach, S., Rugg, D., & et al. (1996). Safer Choices: A multicomponent school-based HIV/STD and pregnancy prevention program for adolescents. *Journal of School Health, 66*(3), 89–110.

Crockenberg, S. (1987). Predictors and correlates of anger toward and punitive control of toddlers by adolescent mothers. *Child Development, 58*(4), 964–975.

Crnic, K., Greenberg, M., Robinson N., & Ragozin, A. (1983). Maternal stress and social support: Effects on the mother-infant relationship from birth to eighteen months. *American Journal of Orthopsychiatry, 54*, 224–235.

Cutrona, C., Hessling, R.M., Bacon, P.L., & Russell, D.W. (1998) Predictors and correlates of continuing involvement with the baby's father among adolescent mothers. *Journal of Family Psychology, 12*(3), 369–387. (in text now)

Dacey, J., & Travers, J. (2002). Adolescence. In *Human development across the lifespan* (5th Ed., pp. 274–332). McGraw–Hill Publishing: New York.

Danziger, S., & Weinberg, D. H. (1994). The historical record: Trends in family income, inequality, and poverty. In S. H. Danziger, G.D. Sandefur, & D.H. Weinberg (Eds.), *Confronting poverty: Prescriptions for change* (pp. 18–50). Cambridge: Harvard University Press,

Darroch, J. E., Landry, D. J., & Oslak, S. (1999). Age differences between sexual partners in the United States. *Family Planning Perspectives, 31*, 160–167.

Darroch, J. E., Landry, D. J., & Singh, S. (2000). Changing emphases in sexuality education in U.S. public secondary schools, 1988–1999. *Family Planning Perspectives, 32*(5).

Davis, E. C., & Friel, L. V. (2001). Adolescent sexuality: disentangling the effects of family structure and family context. *Journal of Marriage and Family, 63*, 669–681.

Dean, A. (1997). *Teenage pregnancy: The interaction of psyche and culture.* Hillsdale, NJ: The Analytic Press.

Deardorf, J., Gonzales, N. A., Christopher, F. S., Roosa, M. S., Milsap, R. E. (2005). Early puberty and adolescent pregnancy: the influence of alcohol use. *Pediatrics, 116*, 1451–1456.

DeCubas, M., & Field, T. (1984). Teaching interactions of black and Cuban teenage mothers and their infants. *Journal of Early Child Development and Care, 16*, 41–56.

Demos, J., & Boocock, S. (1978). *Turning Points: Historical and Sociological Essays on the Family.* Chicago: The University of Chicago Press.

Denny, G., & Young, M. (2006) An evaluation of an abstinence-only sex education curriculum: An 18-month follow-up. *Journal of School Health, 76*(8), 414–422.

Deutsch, H. (19450. *The psychology of women: A psychoanalytic interpretation* (Vol. 2). New York: Grune and Stratton.

Devaney, B., Johnson, A., Maynard, R., & Trenholm, C. (2007). *The evaluation of abstinence education programs funded under Title V Section 510: Interim report.* Princeton, NJ: Mathematica Policy Research, Inc. Contract No: 100-98-0010/MPR Reference No: 8549-110.

DiClemente, R. J., Lodico, M., Grinstead, O. A., Harper, G., Rickman, R. L., Evans, P. E., & et al. (1996). African American adolescents residing in high-risk urban environments do use condoms: Correlates and predictors of condom use among adolescents in a public housing project. *Pediatrics, 98*(2, part 1), 269–278.

DiClemente, R. J., Wingood, G. M., Crosby, G. M., Sinonean, C., Cobb, B., Harrington, K, et al. (2001). Parental monitoring: Association with adolescents' risk behaviors. *Pediatrics, 107*, 1363–1368.

Dilorio, C., Dudley, W. N., Soet, J. E., & McCarty, F. (2004). Sexual possibility situations and sexual behaviors among young adolescents: the moderating role of protective factors. *Journal of Adolescent Health, 35*,528.

Dinerman, L. Wilson, M., Duggan, A., Joffe, A. (1995). Outcomes of adolescents using levonorgestrel implants vs oral contraceptives or other contraceptive methods. *Archives of Pediatric Adolescent Medicine,* *149*, 967–972.

Doniger, A., Adams, E., Utter, C., & Riley, J. (2001). Impact evaluation of the "Not Me, Not Now" abstinence-oriented, adolescent pregnancy prevention communications program, Monroe County, New York. *Journal of Health Communication, 6*, 45–60.

Donnelly, B. W., & Voyandoff, P. (1991). Factors associated with releasing for adoption among adolescent mothers. *Family Relations, 40*, 404–410.

Donovan, P. (1997). Can statutory rape laws be effective in preventing adolescent pregnancy? *Family Planning Perspectives, 29*, 30–34.

Donovan, P. (1999). The "Illegitimacy Bonus" and state efforts to reduce out-of-wedlock births. *Family Planning Perspectives, 31*(2), 94–107.

Drake, St. C., & Cayton, H. (1993;1945). *Black metropolis: A study of Negro life in a northern city.* Chicago: The University of Chicago Press.

Dorius, G., & Baraber, B. (1998). *Parental support and control and the onset of sexual experience.* Unpublished manuscript, Department of Sociology, Brigham Young University, Provo, Utah.

Dryfoos, J. G. (1990). *Adolescents at Risk: Prevalence and Prevention.* New York: Oxford University Press.

Dudley, K. (1939). A referral service for unmarried mothers. *The Family, 20*, 200–202.

Dunbar, J., Sheeder, J., Lezotte, D., Dabelea, D., & Stevens–Simon, C. (2006). Age at menarche and first pregnancy among psychosocially at-risk adolescents. *American Journal of Public Health, 98*(10):1822–1924.

Dworkin, R. J., Harding, J. T., & Schreiber, N. B. (1993). Parenting or placing: Decision making by pregnant teens. *Youth & Society, 25*(1), 75–92.

East, P. L. (1996). Do adolescent pregnancy and childbearing affect younger siblings? *Family Planning Perspectives, 28*(4), 148–153.

East, P. L. (1996) The younger sisters of childbearing adolescents: Their attitudes, expectations, and behaviors. *Child Development, 67*, 267–282.

East, P. L., Felice, M. E., & Morgan, M. C. (1993). Sisters' and girlfriends' sexual and childbearing behavior: effects on early adolescent girls' sexual outcomes. *Journal of Marriage and the Family, 55*, 953–963.

Edin, K. & Lein, L. (1997). *Making ends meet: How single mothers survive welfare and low-wage work.* New York: The Russel Sage Foundation.

Edmunds, L., Rink, E., & Zukoski, A. (2004). Male involvement: Implications for reproductive and sexual health programs. *The Prevention Researcher, 11*, 10–14.

Eisen, M., Pallitto, C., Bradner, C., & Bolshun, N. (2000). *Teen risk-taking: Promising prevention programs and approaches.* Washington, DC: Urban Institute.

Elder, G. (1998). The life course as developmental theory. *Child Development, 69*(1), 1–12.

Elkind, D. (1967). Egocentrism in adolescence. *Child Development, 38*, 1025–1034.

Elkind, D. (1974). *Children and adolescents: Interpretative essay on Jean Piaget.* New York: Oxford University Press.

Elkind, D., & Bowen, R. (1979). Imaginary audience behavior in children and adolescents. *Developmental Psychology, 15*, 38–44.

Elkind, D. (1994). *Ties that stress: The new family imbalance.* Cambridge: Harvard University Press.

Elster, A., McAnarney, E. & Lamb, M. (1983). Parental behavior of adolescent mothers. *Pediatrics, 71,* 494–503.

Emde, R. & Easterbrooks, M. (1985). Assessing emotional availability in early development. In W. K. Frankenburg, R. N. Emde, & J. W. Sullivan (Eds.) *Early identification of children at risk: An international perspective* (pp. 79–101).

Ensminger, M. E. (1987). Adolescent sexual behavior as it relates to other transition behaviors in youth. In S. L. Hofferth & C.D. Hayes (Eds.), *Risking the future: Adolescent sexuality, pregnancy and childbearing, working papers and statistical appendixes.* Washington, DC: National Academy Press.

Erikson, E. (1958). The problems of ego identity. *Journal of American Psychoanalytic Association, 4,* 86–121.

Espeland, K. E. (1997). Inhalants: The instant but deadly high. *Pediatric Nursing, 23*(1), 82–86.

Fagot, B. I., Pears, K. C., Capaldi, D. M., Crosby, L., & Russell, D. W. (1998). Becoming an adolescent father: Precursors and parenting. *Developmental Psychology, 34*(6), 1209–1219.

Farber, N. (1991). The process of pregnancy resolution among adolescent mothers. *Adolescence, 26*(103), 697–716.

Farber, N. (1992). Sexual standards and activity: Adolescents' perceptions. *Child and Adolescent Social Work Journal, 9*(1), 53–76.

Farber, N. (1994). Perceptions of pregnancy risk: A comparison by class and race. *American Journal of Orthopsychiatry, 64*(3), 479–484.

Farber, N. (1999). Teen pregnancy in Wisconsin: Can prevention work? *Wisconsin Policy Research Institute Report, 12*(6), 1–276772.

Farrow, J.A., Watts, D.H., Krohn, M.A., Olson, H.C. (1999). Pregnant adolescents in chemical dependency treatment: Description and outcomes. Journal of Substance Abuse Treatment, Vol 16(2), pp. 157–161.

Federal Register/Vol. 73, No. 24/Tuesday, February 5, 2008/Rules and Regulations.

Field, T., Widmayer, S., Adler, S., & deCubas, M. (1990). Teenage parenting in different cultures, family constellations and caregiving environments: Effects on infant development. *Infant Mental Health Journal, 11*(2), 158–174.

Field, T., Widmayer, S., Stringer, S., & Ignatoff, E. (1980). Teenage, lower-class, black mothers and their preterm infants: An intervention and developmental follow-up. *Child Development, 51,* 426–431.

Fishbein, M. (1997). Predicting, understanding and changing socially relevant behaviors: Lessons learned. In C. McGarty & S.A. Haslam (Eds.). *The Message of Social Psychology* (pp. 77–91). Cambridge, MA: Blackwell Publishers, Inc.

Fishbein, M. (2000). The role of theory in HIV prevention. *AIDS Care, 12*(3), 273–278.

Fisher, G.L. and Harrison, T.C. (2005). Substance Abuse: Information for School Counselors, social workers, therapists, and counselors, 3rd Ed. Boston: Pearson Education.

Flanagan, P., McGrath, M., Meyer, E., & Garcia–Coll, C. (1995). Adolescent development and transitions to motherhood. *Pediatrics, 96,* 273–277.

Focus on young men in pregnancy prevention. (1999). *Contraceptive Technology Update, 20*(8), 92.

Forste, R. T., & Heaton, T. B. (1988). Initiation of sexual activity among female adolescents. *Youth and Society, 19*(3), 250–268.

Fox, G. L., & Inazu, J. K. (1980). Patterns and outcomes of mother-daughter communication about sexuality. *Journal of Social Issues, 36*(1), 7–29.

Fraiberg, S., Adelson, E., & Shapiro, V. (1975). Ghosts in the nursery: A psychoanalytic approach to the problems of impaired infant–mother relationships. *Journal of the American Academy of Child Psychiatry, 14*(3), 387–422.

Fraiberg, S. & Fraiberg, L. (1980). *Clinical studies in infant mental health: The first year of life.* New York: Basic Books.

Frank, D. A., Augustyn, M., Knight, W. G., Pell, T., & Zuckerman, B. (2001). Growth, development, and behavior in early childhood following prenatal cocaine exposure: A systematic review. *Journal of the American Medical Association, 285,* 1613–1625.

Franklin, D. (1988). Race, class, and adolescent pregnancy: An ecological analysis. *American Journal of Orthopsychiatry, 58*(3), 339–338.

Fraser, M. (1997). *Risk and resilience in childhood: An ecological perspective.* Washington, DC: NASW Press.

Frazier, E. F. (1939). *The Negro Family in the United States.* Chicago: The University of Chicago Press.

Frazier, E. F. (1957). *Black Bourgeoisie.* Toronto, Ontario: MacMillan Company.

Freeman, E. M. (1987). Interaction of pregnancy, loss and developmental issues in adolescents. *Social Casework* (January 1987), 38–46.

Freud, A. (1965). Normality and pathology of development in childhood: Assessments of development. New York: International Universities Press.

Freud, A. (1968). Adolescence. In A.E. Winder & D. L. Angus (Eds.), *Adolescence: Contemporary studies.* New York: American Book.

Frost, J. J., & Forrest, J. D. (1995). Understanding the impact of effective teenage pregnancy prevention programs. *Family Planning Perspectives, 27,* 188–195.

Furstenberg, F. (1976). *Unplanned Parenthood: The Social Consequences of Teenage Childbearing.* New York: The Free Press.

Furstenberg, F., Brooks–Gunn, J., & Levine, J. (1990). The children of teenage mothers: Patterns of early childbearing in two generations. *Family Planning Perspectives, 22,* 54–61.

Furstenberg, F. F., Brooks–Gunn, J., & Morgan, P. S. (1987). *Adolescent Mothers Later in Life.* Cambridge: Cambridge University Press.

Furstenberg, F. F. (2007). *Destinies of the disadvantaged.* New York: Russell Sage Foundation.

Government Accountability Office (GAO). (2006). *Abstinence Education: Efforts to Assess the Accuracy and Effectiveness of Federally Funded Programs.* Washington, DC: United States Government Accountability Office. GAO-07-87.

Garcia–Coll, C., Hoffman, J., & Oh, W. (1987). The social context of teenage childbearing: Effects on the infant's caregiving environment. *Journal of Youth and Adolescence, 16,* 345–360.

Gibbs, L. T., & Huang, L. N. (1999) (Eds.). *Children of color: Psychological interventions with culturally diverse youth.* California: Jossey–Bass.

Gibson, J. W., & Kempf, J. (1990). Attitudinal predictors of sexual activity in Hispanic adolescent females. *Journal of Adolescent Research, 5*(4), 414–430.

Glei, D. A. (1999). Measuring contraceptive use patterns among teenage and adult women. *Family Planning Perspectives, 31*, 73–80.

Gold, R. B. (2000). Adolescent care standards and state CHIP efforts. *The Guttmacher Report on Public Policy.* New York: The Alan Guttmacher Institute.

Gold, R. B. (2001). Title X: Three decades of accomplishment. *The Guttmacher Report on Policy.* New York: The Alan Guttmacher Institute.

Gold, R., Connell, F., Haegerty, P., Cummings, P., Bezruchka, S., Davis, R., et al. (2005). Predicting time to subsequent pregnancy. *Maternal and Child Health Journal, 9*(3), 219–226.

Goode, W. (1961). Illegitimacy, *anomie and cultural penetration. American Sociological* Review, *28*(6), 910–925.

Goodson, P., Pruitt, B., Suther, S., Wilson, K., & Buhi, E. (2006). Is abstinence education theory based? The underlying logic of abstinence education programs in Texas. *Health Education and Behavior, 33*(2), 252–271.

Gordon, C. P. (1996). Adolescent decision making: A broadly based theory and its application to the prevention of early pregnancy. *Adolescence, 31*, 561–584.

Grady, W. R., Hayward, M. D., & Billy, J. O. G. (1989). *A dynamic model of premarital pregnancy in the U.S.* Final report to the office of population affairs, U.S. Department of Health and Human Services. Seattle, WA: Battell Human Affairs Research Centers.

Greenberg, M. S., Singh, T., Htoo, M., & Schultz, S. (1991). The association between congenital syphilis and cocaine/crack cocaine use in New York City: A case-control study. *American Journal of Public Health, 81*, 1316–131.

Greenberg, P. (1989). Parents as partners in young children's development and education: A new American fad? Why does it matter? *Young Children,* May, 61–75.

Grotevant, H., & Cooper, C. (1986). Individuation in family relationships: A perspective on individual differences in the development of identity and role-taking skill in adolescence. *Human Development, 29*, 82–100.

Guilamo–Ramos, V., Jaccard, J., Dittus, P., Gonzalez, B., & Bouris, A. (2008). A conceptual framework for the analysis of risk and problem behaviors: The case of adolescent sexual behavior." *Social Work, 32*(1), 29–44.

Guttmacher Institute. (2006a). *Facts on sex education in the United States.*

Guttmacher Institute. (2006b). *U.S. Teenage Pregnancy Statistics.* New York: Guttmacher Institute.

Guttmacher Institute State Policies in Brief. (2008a). *Sex and STI/HIV Education.*

Guttmacher Institute State Policies in Brief. (2008b). *Parental Involvement in Minors' Abortions.*

Guttmacher Institute State Policies in Brief. (2008c). *Minors' Access to Prenatal Care.*

Guttmacher Institute Policies in Brief. (2008d). *An Overview of Minors' Consent Law.*

Guttmachaer Institute Policies in Brief. (2008e). *Minors' Access to Contraceptive Services.*

Guttmacher Institute State Policies in Brief. (2008f). *Minors' Rights as Parents.*

Guttmacher Institute. (2008g). *Facts on Publicly Funded Contraceptive Services.* Retrieved October 20, 2008, from http://www. guttmacher. org/pubs/fb_contraceptive_serv.html.

Halpern, C. T., Joyner, K., Udry, R., & Suchindran, C. (2000). Smart teens don't have sex (or kiss much). *Journal of Adolescent Health, 26*(3), 213–225.

Hamilton, G. (1923). Progress in social case work. *The Family, 4*(5), 111–118.

Hamilton, B. E., Martin, J. A., & Ventura, S, J. (2007). Births: Preliminary data for 2006. *CDC National Vital Statistics Reports, 56*(7).

Harari, S. E., & Vinovskis, M. A. (1993). Adolescent sexuality, pregnancy, and childbearing in the past. In A. E. Lawson & D.L. Rhode (Eds.), *The politics of pregnancy* (pp. 23–45). New Haven: Yale University Press.

Hatcher, S. (1976). Understanding adolescent pregnancy and abortion. *Primary Care, 3,* 407–425.

Hawkins, J. D., Catalano, R. F., Kosterman, R., Abbott, R., & Hill, K. G. (1999). Preventing adolescent health-risk behaviors by strengthening protection during childhood. *Archives of Pediatrics and Adolescent Medicine, 153*(3), 226–234.

Hayes, C. D. (1987). *Risking the future: Adolescent sexuality, pregnancy, and childbearing.* Washington, DC: National Academy Press.

Herman–Giddens, M., Kaplowitz, P., & Wasserman, R., (2004). Navigating the recent articles on girls' puberty in pediatrics: What do we know and where do we go from here? *Pediatrics, 113*(4), 911–917.

Hill, J. (1987). Central changes during adolescence. In W. Damon (Ed.), *New directions in child psychology.* San Francisco: Jossey–Bass.

Hodgins, D. C., El–Guebaly, N., & Addington, J. (1997). Treatment of substance abusers: Single or mixed gender programs? *Addiction, 92*(7), 805–812.

Hoff, T., McIntosh, M., Rawlings, N., & D'Amico, J. (2000). *Sex education in America: Summary of findings.* Menlo Park, CA: Henry J. Kaiser Family Foundation.

Hofferth, S. (1987). The effects of programs and policies on adolescent pregnancy and childbearing. In C. Hayes, (Ed.), *Risking the future.* (Vol 1). Washington, DC: National Academy Press.

Hoffman, S. (2006). *By the numbers: The public costs of teen childbearing.* Washington, DC: The National Campaign to Prevent Teen Pregnancy.

Hoffman, S., & Maynard, R. (2008). *Kids having kids.* Washington, DC: The Urban Institute Press.

Hogan, D. P., & Kitagawa, E. M. (1985). The impact of social status, family structure, and neighborhood on the fertility of black adolescents. *American Journal of Sociology, 90*(4), 825–855.

Hopkins, K. R. (1987). *Welfare dependency: Behavior, culture and public policy.* U.S. Department of Health and Human Services, Contract No. 100-86-0022.

Horner, J. R., Carey, M. P., Vanable, P., Salazar, L., Carey, M., Juzang, I., et al. (2008). Using culture-centered qualitative formative research to design broadcasts messages for HIV-prevention for African American adolescents. *Journal of Health Communication, 13*(4), 309–325.

Horowitz, N.H. (1978). Adolescent mourning reactions to infant and fetal loss. *Social Casework*, 551–559.

Horrigan, T. J., Schroeder, A. V., & Schaffer, R. M. (2000). The triad of substance abuse, violence, and depression are interrelated in pregnancy. *Journal of Substance Abuse Treatment, 18*(1), 55–59.

Hovell, M., Sipan, C., Blumberg, E., Atkins, C., Hofstetter, C. R., & Kreitner, S. (1994). Family influences on Latino and Anglo adolescents' sexual behavior. *Journal of Marriage and the Family, 56*, 973–986.

Howell, E. M., Heiser, N., & Harrington, M. (1999). *Journal of Substance Abuse Treatment, 16*(3), 195–219.

Hubbs-Tait, L., Hughes, K., Culp, A., Osofsky, J., Hann, D., Eberhart-Wright, A., & Ware, L. (1996). Children of adolescent mothers: Attachment representations, maternal depression, and later behavior problems. *American Journal of Orthopsychiatry, 66*, 416–426.

Huebner, A. J., & Howell, L. W. (2003). Examining the relationship between adolescent sexual risk-taking and perceptions of monitoring, communication and parenting styles. *Journal of Adolescent Health, 33*, 71–78.

Huizinga, D., Loeber, R., & Thornberry, T. P. (1993). Longitudinal study of delinquency, drug use, sexual activity, and pregnancy among children and youth in three cities. *Public Health Reports, 108*, 90–97.

Humphries, D. (1999). Crack mothers: Pregnancy, Drugs and the Media. Columbus, OH: Ohio State University press.

Inazu, J. K., & Fox, G. L. (1980). Maternal influences on the sexual behavior of teen-age daughters: Direct and indirect sources. *Journal of Family Issues, 1*(1), 81–102.

Inciardi, J. A., Lockwood, D., & Potttieger, A. E. (1992). *Women and Crack cocaine*. New York: McMillan.

Institute of Medicine. (1996). *Fetal alcohol syndrome: Diagnosis, epidemiology, prevention, and treatment*. Washington, DC: National Academy Press.

Iversen, R. R., & Farber, N. (1999). Transmission of family values, work and welfare among poor urban black women. In T.L Parcel & D.B. Cornfield (Eds.). *Work and family: Research informing policy* (pp. 249–274). Thousand Oaks: Sage Publications, Inc.

Jaccard, J., & Dittus, P. (1991). *Parent-teen Communication: Toward the Prevention of unintended pregnancies*. New York: Springer–Verlag.

Jaccard, J., Dittus, P. J., & Gordon, V. V. (1996). Maternal correlates of adolescent sexual and contraceptive behavior. *Family Planning Perspectives, 28*, 159–165, 185.

Jenson, J. M., Howard, M. O., & Yaffe, J. (1995). Treatment of adolescent substance abusers: Issues for practice and research. *Social Work in Health Care, 21*(2), 1–18.

Jessor, S., & Jessor, R. (1975). Transition from virginity to nonvirginity among youth: A social–psychological study over time. *Developmental Psychology, 11*(11), 47–484.

Jessor, S., & Jessor, R. (1977). *Problem behavior and psychological development: A longitudinal study of youth*. New York: Academic Press.

Johns, M., Moncloa, F., & Gong, E. (2000). Teen pregnancy prevention: Linking research and practice. *Journal of Extension*. Retrieved September 19, 2008, from http://www.joe.org/joe/2000august/a1.html.

Josselson, R. (1987). *Finding herself: Pathways to identity development in women*. San Francisco: Jossey–Bass, Inc.

Juster, S.M., & M.A. Vinovskis. (1987). Changing perspectives on the American family in the past. *Annual Review of Sociology, 13*, 193–216.

Kahn, J. G., Brindis, C., & Glei, D. A. (1999). Pregnancies averted among U.S. teenagers by the use of contraceptives. *Family Planning Perspectives, 31*, 29–34.

Kalmuss, D., & Namerow, P. (1994). Subsequent childbearing among teenage mothers: The determinants of a closely spaced second birth. *Family Planning Perspectives, 26*(4), 149–159.

Kastsner, L.S., (1984). Ecological factors predicting adolescent contraceptive use: Implications for intervention. *Journal of Adolescent Health Care, 5*(2), 79–86.

KFF – The Henry J. Kaiser Family Foundation. (2000). *Teen sexual activity. Fact Sheet*. Retrieved September 18, 2008, from http://www.kff.org.

KFF – The Henry J. Kaiser Family Foundation. (2001). *Trends in CHIP expenditures: State-by-state data*. The Kaiser Commission on Medicaid and the Uninsured. Menlo Park: The Henry J. Kaiser Family Foundation.

KFF – The Henry J. Kaiser Family Foundation. (2005). U.S. Teen Sexual Activity, http://www.kff.org/youthhivstds/upload/U-S-Teen-Sexual-Activity-Fact-Sheet.pdf

Keefe, M. (2007). *Abstinence-only-until-marriage programs: Ineffective, unethical, and poor public health*. Washington, D.C.: Advocates for Youth

Kirby, D. (2001). *No easy answers: Research findings on programs to reduce teen pregnancy*. Washington, DC: National Campaign to Prevent Teen Pregnancy.

Kirby, D. (2004). *BDI Logic models: A useful tool for designing, strengthening and evaluating programs to reduce adolescent risk-taking, pregnancy, HIV and other STDs*. Retrieved September 1, 2008, from http://www.etr.org.recapp/lBDILOGICMODEL20630924.pdf.

Kirby, D. (2007). Emerging answers 2007: *Research findings on programs to reduce teen pregnancy and sexually transmitted diseases*. Washington, DC: National Campaign to Prevent Teen Pregnancy.

Kirby, D., Denner, J., & Coyle, K. (2000). *Building the ideal community or youth program: An expert panel rates the key characteristics for reducing teen pregnancy*. Washington, DC: National Campaign to Prevent Teen Pregnancy.

Kissman, K., & Shapiro, J. (1990). The composites of social support and well-being among adolescent mothers. *International Journal of Adolescence and Youth, 2*, 165–173.

Klerman, L. (2004). *Another chance: Preventing additional births to teen mothers*. Washington, DC: National Campaign to Prevent Teen Pregnancy.

Knight, J. R., Goodman, E., Pulerwitz, T., & DuRant, R. H. (2000). Reliabilities of short substance abuse screening tests among adolescent medical patients. *Pediatrics, 105*(4, Pt 2), 948–953.

Kolodny, R. L., & Reilly, W. V. (1972). Group work with today's unmarried mother. *Social Casework,* 613–622.

Kokotailo, P. K., Adger, H., Duggan, A. K., Repke, J., & Joffe, Alain. (1992). Cigarette, alcohol, and other drug use by school-age pregnant adolescents: Prevalence, detection, and associated high risk factors. *Pediatrics, 90*(3), 328–334.

Koniak–Griffin, D., & Brecht, M. L. (1995). Linkages between sexual risk taking, substance use, and AIDS knowledge among pregnant adolescents and young mothers. *Nursing Research, 44*(6), 340–346.

Kroger, J. (2000). *Identity development: Adolescence through adulthood.* California: Sage Publications.

Ku, L., Sonenstein, F. L., & Pleck, J. H. (1993a). Factors influencing first intercourse for teenage men. *Public Health Reports, 108*(6), 680–694.

Ku, L., Sonenstein, F. L., & Pleck, J. H. (1993b). Neighborhood, family, and work: Influences on premarital behaviors of adolescent males. *Social Forces, 72*(2), 479–503.

Ladner, J. (1971). *Tomorrow's tomorrow: The Black women.* Garden City, NY: Doubleday & Co.

Lammers, C., Ireland, M., Resnick, M., & Blum, R. (2000). Influences on adolescents' decision to postpone onset of sexual intercourse: A survival analysis of virginity among youths aged 13–18 years. *Journal of Adolescent Health, 26*(1), 42–48.

Lancaster, J. B., & Hamburg, B. A. (1986). *School-age pregnancy and parenthood: Biosocial dimensions.* New York: Aldine De Gruyter.

Landy, S. (1984). The individuality of teenage mothers and its implications for intervention strategies. *Journal of Adolescence, 7,* 171–290.

Landry, D. J., Kaeser, L., & Richards, C. L. (1999). Abstinence promotion and the provision of information about contraception in public school district sexuality education policies. *Family Planning Perspectives, 31*(6), 280–286.

Lapsley, D.K. (1993). The two faces of adolescent invulnerability. In D. Romer (Ed.), *Reducing adolescent adolescent risk: Toward an integrated approach* (pp. 25–32). Thousand Oaks, CA: Sage Publications, Inc.

Latimer, W. W., Newcomb, M., Winters, K. C., & Stinchfield, R. D. (2000). Adolescent substance abuse treatment outcome: The role of substance abuse problem severity, psychosocial, and treatment factors. *Journal of Consulting and Clinical Psychology, 68*(4), 684–696.

Lauritsen, J. L. (1994) Explaining race and gender differences in adolescent sexual behavior. *Social Forces, 72*(3), 859–883.

Lauritsen, J. L., & Swicegood, C. G. (1997). The consistency of self-reported initiation of sexual activity. *Family Planning Perspectives, 29*(5), 215–221.

LeCroy and Milligan Associates, Inc. (2003). *Final report: Arizona abstinence only education.* Tuscon, AZ: LeCroy and Milligan Associates, Inc.

Levine, L., Garcia Coll, C., & Oh, W. (1975). Determinants of mother-infant interaction in adolescent mothers. *Journal of the American Academy of Child and Adolescent Psychiatry, 24*(3), 374.

Lewis, O. (1965). *La vida*. New York: Vintage Books.

Li, X., Feigelman, S., & Stanton, B. (2000). Perceived parental monitoring and health risk behaviors among urban low-income African-American children and adolescents. *Journal of Adolescent Health, 27*, 43–48.

Liddle, H. A. (1992). Family therapy techniques for adolescents with drug and alcohol problems. In W. Snyder & T. Ooms (Eds.), *Empowering families* (ADAMHA Monograph from the First National Conference on the Treatment of Adolescent Drug, Alcohol and Mental Health Problems). Washington, DC: United States Public Health Service, U. S. Government Printing Office.

Lieberman, F. (1973). Sex and the adolescent girl: liberation or exploitation? Clinical *Social Work Journal, 1*(4), 224–243.

Liebow, E. (1967). *Tally's corner*. Boston: Little, Brown and Company.

Little, R. (1944). Consultation service for girls with venereal disease. *The Family: Journal of Social Casework, 225*(5), 163–169.

Longmore, M. S., Manning, W. D., & Giordano, P. C. (2001). Preadolescent parenting strategies and teens' dating and sexual initiation: A longitudinal analysis. *Journal of Marriage and the Family, 63*, 322–335.

Low cost health insurance for families and children. (n.d.). Retrieved April 14, 2009, from http://www.cms.hhs.gov/LowCostHealthInsFamChild/

Luker, K. (1996). *Dubious conceptions: The politics of teenage pregnancy*. Cambridge, MA: Harvard University Press.

Malinowski, B. (1930). Parenthood: The basis of social structure. In Culverton, V. & Schmalhousen (Eds.), *The new generation*. New York: Macauley.

Manlove, J., Mariner, C., & Papillo, A. (2000). Subsequent fertility among teen mothers: Longitudinal analyses of recent national data. *Journal of Marriage and Family, 62*, 430–448.

Manlove, J., Ryan, S., & Franzetta, K. (2007). Contraceptive use patterns across teens' sexual relationships: The role of relationships, partners, and sexual histories. *Demography, 44*(3): 603–621.

Marcia, J. E. (1994). The empirical study of ego identity. In H. Bosma & T. Graafsma (Eds.), *Identity and development: An interdisciplinary approach* (pp. 67–80). California: Sage Publications.

Marin, B. V., Coyle, K. K., Gomez, C. A., Carvajal, S. C., & Kirby, D. B. (2000). Older boyfriends and girlfriends increase risk of sexual initiation in young adolescents. *Journal of Adolescent Health, 27*(6), 409–418.

Martin, J. A., Hamilton, B. E., Sutton, P. D., Ventura, S. J., Menacker, F., Kirmeyer, S., et al 2007). Birth: Final data for 2005. *National Vital Statistics Reports 2007, 56*(6).

Martin, J. A., Hamilton, B. E., Sutton, P. D., & Ventura, S. J. (2009). *Births: Final data for 2006*. National Vital Statistics Reports; vol 57 no 7. Hyattsville, MD: National Center for Health Statistics.

Masten, A. S., Hubbard, J., Gest, S., Tellegen, A., & Garmezy, N. (1999). Competence in the context of adversity: Pathways to resilience and maladaptation from childhood to late adolescence. *Development and Psychopathology, 11*(1), 143–169.

Masters, T., Beadnell, B., & Hoppe, M. (2008). The opposite of sex? Adolescents' thoughts about abstinence and sex, and their sexual behavior. *Perspectives on Sexual and Reproductive Health, 40*(2), 87–93.

Maynard, R., Trenholm, C., Devaney, B., Johnson, A., Clark, M., Homrighausen, J., et al. (2005). *First-year impacts of four Title V, Section 510 abstinence education programs*. Princeton, NJ: Mathematica Policy, Inc. Contract No: HHS 100-98-0010/MPR Reference No: 8549-110.

McAnarney, E. (1983). *Premature adolescent pregnancy and parenthood.* New York: Grune and Stratton.

McLanahan, S., & Sandefur, G. (1994). *Growing up with a single parent: What hurts, what helps.* Cambridge, MA: Harvard University Press.

Mendea–Netgrete, J., Saldana, & Vega, A. (2006). Can a culturally informed after-school curriculum make a difference in teen pregnancy prevention? Preliminary Evidence in the case of San Antonio's Escuelitas. *Families in Society, 87*(1), 95–104.

Mercer, R. (1986). Teenage motherhood: The first year. *JOGN Nursing, 9*, 16–22.

Miller, C., Miceli, P., Whitman, T., & Borkowski, J. (1996). Cognitive readiness to parent and intellectual-emotional development in children of adolescent mothers. *Developmental Psychology, 32*(3), 533–541.

Miller, B. C., Card, J. J., Paikoff, R. L., & Peterson, J. L. (1992). *Preventing adolescent pregnancy: Model programs and evaluations.* Newbury Park: Sage Publications.

Miller, B. C. (1998). *Families matter: A research synthesis of family influences on adolescent pregnancy.* Washington, D.C: National Campaign to Prevent Teen Pregnancy.

Miller, K. S., Forehand, R., & Kotchick, B. A. (1999). Adolescent sexual behavior in two ethnic minority samples: The role of family variables. *Journal of Marriage and the Family, 61*, 85–98.

Miller, K. S., Forehand, R., & Kitchick, B. A. (2000). Adolescent sexual behavior in two ethnic minority groups: a multisystem perspective. *Adolescence, 138*, 313–333.

Moffitt, R. (1992). Incentive effects of the U.S. welfare system: A review. *Journal of Economic Literature, 30*, 1–61.

Monahan, D. (2001). Teen pregnancy prevention outcomes: Implications for social work practice. *Families in Society, 82*(2), 127–135.

Moon, E. (1998). Pregnant, hooked & booked. *Professional Counselor,* 13–16.

Moore, K., & Caldwell, S. B. (1977). *Out-of-wedlock childbearing.* Washington, DC: Urban Institute, Mimeographed.

Moore, K., Morrison, D. R., & Glei, D. A. (1995). Welfare and adolescent sex: The effects of family history, benefit levels, and community context. *Journal of Family and Economic Issues, 16*, 207–237.

Moore, M. R., & Chase-Lansdale, P. L. (1999). Sexual intercourse and pregnancy among African American adolescent girls in high-poverty neighborhoods: The role of family and perceived community environment. Unpublished draft.

Moore, K., & Snyder, N. (1990). *Cognitive development among the children of adolescent mothers.* Washington, DC: Child Trends.

Moore, K., & Sugland, B. (1997). Using behavioral theories to design abstinence programs. *Children and Youth Services Review, 19*(5,6), 485–500.

Moore, K. (2008). Teen births: Examining the recent increase. Washington, DC: The National Campaign to Prevent Teen and Unplanned Pregnancy.

Morgan, E. S. (1983). Puritans and sex. In M. Gordon (Ed.), *The American family in social-historical perspective* (pp. 311–320). New York: S. Martins Press

Mott, F. L., & Jaurin, R. J. (1988). Linkages between sexual activity and alcohol and drug use among American adolescents. *Family Planning Perspectives, 27*, 18–22, 33.

Murray, C. (1984). *Losing ground.* New York: Basic Books, Inc., Pub.

Muck, R., Zempolich, K.A., Titus, J.C., Fishman, M., Godley, M.D., & Schwebel, R. Special issue: Bringing restorative justice to adolescent substance abuse. Youth & Society, Vol 33(2), 143–168.

Muck, R., Zempolich, K.A., Titus, J., Fishman, M. Godley, M. D., & Schwebel, R. (2001). An overview of the effectiveness of adolescent substance abuse treatment models. *Youth and Society, 33*(2), 143–168.

Musick, J. S. (1993). *Young, poor, and pregnant: The psychology of teenage motherhood.* New Haven: Yale University Press.

Musick, J., & Stott, S. (2000). In Shonkoff, J. & Meisels (Eds.), Handbook of early childhood intervention. (pp. 349–353). Cambridge, UK: Cambridge University Press.

Nagy, S., DiClemente, R. J., & Adcock, A. G. (1995). Adverse factors associated with forced sex among southern adolescent girls. *Pediatrics, 96*, 944–946.

Nath, P., Borkowski, J., Whitman, T., & Schellenbach, C. (1991). Understanding adolescent parenting: The dimensions and functions of social support. *Family Relations, 40*: 411–419.

Nathan, R. P., Gentry, P., & Lawrence, C. (1999). *Is there a link between welfare reform and teen pregnancy? Rockefeller Reports.* Albany, NY: The Nelson A. Rockefeller Institute of Government.

National Campaign to Prevent Teen Pregnancy. (1999a). *Get Organized: A guide to preventing teen pregnancy.* Washington, DC: The National Campaign to Prevent Teen Pregnancy.

National Campaign to Prevent Teen Pregnancy (1999b). *Fact sheet: Teen pregnancy and childbearing among Latinos in the United States.* Washington, DC: National Campaign to Prevent Teen Pregnancy. Retrieved October 1, 2008 from http://www.teenpregnnacy.org/fact_latam.htm.

National Campaign to Prevent Teen Pregnancy. (2001). In H. Cothran (Ed.), *Teen pregnancy is a serious problem.* In Teen Pregnancy and Parenting (pp.18–23). San Diego: Greenhaven Press, Inc.

National Campaign to Prevent Teen Pregnancy. (2000). *Facts and Stats*[Online]. Available at: http://www.teenpregnancy.org/genlfact.htm. Accessed July 5, 2000.

National Council of Family and Juvenile Court Judges (1987). *Juvenile and family substance abuse: A judicial response.* Reno, NV: National Council of Family Court Judges.

Neinstein, L. S., Gordon, C. M., Katzman, D. K., Rosen, D. S., & Woods, E. R. (2009). *Adolescent Healthcare: A practical guide.* (5th ed). Philadelphia: Lippincott Williams & Wilkins.

Nelson–Zlupko, L., Kauffman, E., & Dore, M. M. (1995). Gender differences in drug addiction and treatment: implications for social work intervention with substance-abusing women. *Social Work, 40*(1), 45–54.

Neuspiel, D. R., Zingman, T. M., Templeton, V. H., DiStabile, P., & Drucker, E.(1993). Custody of cocaine-exposed newborns: Determinants of discharge decisions. *American Journal of Public Health, 83*, 1726–1729.

Newcomer, S., & Udry, J. R. (1987). Parental marital status effects on adolescent sexual behavior. *Journal of Marriage and the Family, 49*, 235–240.

Office of Population Affairs. *Title XX overview*. Available at: http://www.hhs.gov/progorg.opa/titlexx/oapp.html. Retrieved December 1, 2000.

Office of Population Affairs. *Title XX: Adolescent family life demonstration projects. Text of findings and purposes*. Available:http://opa.osophs.dhhs.gov/titlexx/xxstatut.txt. Retrieved October 8, 2001.

Ohannesian, C., & Crockett, L. (1993). A longitudinal investigation of the relationship between educational investment and adolescent sexual activity. *Journal of Adolescent Research, 8*(2), 167–182.

Osofsky, J., Eberhart–Wright, A., Ware, L., & Hann, D. (1992). Children of adolescent mothers: A group at risk for psychopathology. *Infant Mental Health Journal, 13*(2), 119–131.

O'Sullivan, L. F., & Brooks-Gunn, J. (2005). The timing of changes in girls' sexual cognitions and behaviors in early adolescence: a prospective, cohort study. *Journal of Adolescent Health, 68*(8), 334–338.

Pagliaro, A. M., & Paglianro, L. A. (2000). *Substance use among women*. Philadelphia: Brunner/Mazel.

Perkins, D. F., Luster, T., Villarruel, F. A., & Small, S. (1998). An ecological, risk-factor examination of adolescents' sexual activity in three ethnic groups. *Journal of Marriage and Family, 60*, 660–673.

Perlman, H. H. (1957). *Social casework: A problem-solving process*. Chicago: The University of Chicago Press.

Perlman, H. H. (1964). An approach to social work problems: Perspectives of the unmarried mother on AFDC. Presentation at the Meeting of State Welfare Leadership Staff on Program Development of Social Services, Bureau of Family Services, Welfare Administration, Department of Health, Education and Welfare, July 6–10, 1964, Washington, DC.

Piazza, N. J., Martin, N., Dildine, R.J. (2000). Screening instruments for alcohol and other drug problems. Journal of Mental Health Counseling, Vol 22(3), pp. 218–227.

Piccinino, L. J., & Mosher, W. D. (1998). Trends in contraceptive use in the United States: 1982–1995. *Family Planning Perspectives, 30*, 4–10.

Pick, S., & Palos, P. A. (1995). Impact of the family on the sex lives of adolescents. *Adolescence, 30*, 667–675.

PPF – Planned Parenthood Federation of America, Inc. (2000). *Reducing teenage pregnancy*. Fact Sheet, Planned Parenthood Web Site. Retrieved August 8, 2008, from http://www.plannedparenthood.org/library/TEEN-PREGNANCY/Reducing.html.

Pope, S., Whiteside, L., Brooks–Gunn, J., Kelleher, K., Rickert, V., Bradley, R. et al. (1993). Low-birthweight infants born to adolescent mothers: Effects of coresidency with grandmother on child development. *JAMA, 269*(11): 1396–1400.

Quinn, W., Newfield, N., & Protinsky, H. (1985). Rites of passage in families with adolescents. *Family Processes, 24*, 101–111.

Radin, N., Oyserman, D., & Benn, R. (1990). *Grandfather influence on the young children of teenage mothers*. Paper presented at the Biennial Meeting of the Society for Research on Child Development. Kansas City, MO. April.

Ragozin, A., Basham, R., Crnic, K., Greenberg, N., & Robinson, N. (1982). Effects of maternal age on parenting role. *Developmental Psychology, 18*, 627–634.

Raine. T. R., Jenkins, R., Aarons, S. J., Woodwarwd, K., Fairfax, J. L., El-Khorazaty, M. N., et al. (1999). Sociodemographic correlates of virginity in seventh-grade black and Latino students. *Journal of Adolescent Health, 24*(5), 304–312.

Rains, P. (1971). *Becoming an unwed mother*. Chicago: Aldine Pub. Co.

Rainwater, L. (1970). *Behind Ghetto walls: Black families in a federal slum*. Chicago: Aldine Publishing Co.

Rall, M. E. (1947). Dependency and the adolescent. *Journal of Social Casework, 47,*123–130.

Ramirez–Valles, J., Zimmerman, M. A., & Juarez, L. (2002). Gender differences of neighborhood and social control processes: A study of the timing of first intercourse among low-achieving, urban, African American youth. *Youth Society, 33*(3):418–441.

Rao, U., Daley, S. E., & Hammen, C. Relationship between depression and substance use disorders in adolescent women during the transition to adulthood. *Journal of the American Academy of Child and Adolescent Psychiatry, 39*(2), 215–222.

Ravoira, L., & Cherry, A. L. (1992). *Social bonds and teen pregnancy*. Westport, CT: Praeger.

Raymond, M., Bogdanovich, Brahmi, D., Cardinal, L. J., Fager, G. L., Fratterelli, L., et al. (2008). State refusal of federal funding for abstinence-only programs. *Sexuality Research and Social Policy, 5*(3): 44–44.

Ream, G. L., & Savin–Williams, R. C., (2005). Reciprocal associations between adolescent sexual activity and quality of youth–parent interactions. *Journal of Family Psychology, 19*(2);171–179.

Resnick, M. D. (1984). Studying adolescent mothers' decision making about adoption and parenting. *Social Work*, 5–10.

Resnick, M.D., Bearman, P.S., Blum, R.W., Bauman, K.E., Harris, K.M., Jones, J., et al. (1997). Protecting adolescents from harm: Findings from the National Longitudinal Study on Adolescent Health. *Journal of American Medical Association, 278*(10), 823–832.

Roberts, R. (1966). *The unwed mother*. New York: Harper & Row Pub.

Rodman, H. (1971). Lower-class families: The culture of poverty in Negro Trinidad. New York: Oxford University Press.

Rome, R. (1940). A method of predicting the probable dispositions of their children by unmarried mothers. *Smith College Studies in Social Work, 10*(3), 167–201.

Romer, D., Stanton, B., Galbraith, J., Feigelman, S., Black, M., & Li, X. (1999). Parental influence on adolescent sexual behavior in high-poverty settings. *Archives of Pediatric Adolescent Medicine, 153*(10), 1055062.

Roosa, M. W., Tein, J. Y., Reingholtz, C., & Angelini, P. J. (1997). The relationship of childhood sexual abuse to teenage pregnancy. *Journal of Marriage and the Family, 59*, 119–130.

Root, M.P. (1989). Treatment failures: The role of victimization in women's addictive behavior. American Journal of Orthopsychiatry, 59(4 Oct.), 542–549.

Rose, A., Koo, H. P., Bhaskar, B., et al. (2005). The influence of primary caregivers on the sexual behavior of early adolescents. *Journal of Adolescent Health, 37*, 135–144.

Rosenbaum, E., & Kandel, D.B. (1990). Early onset of adolescent sexual behavior and drug involvement. *Journal of Marriage and the Family, 52*, 783–798.

Rosenthal, S. L., Von Ranson, K. M., Cotton, S., et al. (2001). Sexual initiation: Predictors and developmental trends. *Sexual Transmission of Disease, 28*(9), 527–532.

Roye, C., & Hudson, M. (2003). Development of a culturally appropriate video to promote dual method use by urban teens: Rationale and methodology. *AIDS Education Prevention,* 15, 148–158.

Sabo, D. F., Miller, K. E., Farrell, M. P., Melnick, M. J., & Barnes, G. M. (1999). High school athletic participation, sexual behavior and adolescent pregnancy: A regional study. *Journal of Adolescent Health, 25*, 207–216.

Sadler, L., & Catrone, C. (1983). The adolescent parent: A dual developmental crisis. *Journal of Adolescent Health Care, 4*, 100–105.

Saleeaby, D. (1997). *The strengths perspective in social work practice*. (2nd ed.). New York: Longman.

Sangalang, B., & Rounds, K. (2005). Differences in health behaviors and parenting knowledge between pregnant adolescents and parenting adolescents. *Social Work in Health Care, 42*, 21–23.

Sangalang, B., Barth, R., & Painter, J. (2006). First-birth outcomes and timing of second births: A statewide case management program for adolescent mothers. *Health and Social Work, 31*(1), 54–64.

Santelli, J. S., Lowry, R., Brener, N. D., & Robin, L. (2000). The association of sexual behaviors with socioeconomic status, family structure, and race/ethnicity among US adolescents. *American Journal of Public Health, 90*, 1582–1587.

Sather, L., & Zinn, K. (2002). Effects of abstinence-only education on adolescent attitudes and values concerning premarital sexual intercourse. *Family Community Health, 25*(2), 1–15.

Sawhill, I., & Hutchins, J. (2000). *Investing welfare funds in teen pregnancy prevention*. Washington, DC: National Campaign to Prevent Teen Pregnancy.

Schaeffer, C., & Pine, F. (1972). Pregnancy, abortion, and the developmental tasks of adolescence. *Journal of the American Academy of Child Psychiatry, 11*, 511–536.

Schamess, G. (1991). Toward an understanding of the etiology and treatment of psychological dysfunction among single teenage mothers. *Journal of Smith College School of Social Work, 60*, 143–175.

Scherz, F. H. (1947). "Taking sides" in the unmarried mother's conflict. *Journal of Social Casework, 28*, 47–61.

Schinke, S. (1978) Adolescent pregnancy: An interpersonal skill training approach to prevention. *Social Work in Health Care, 3*, 159–167.

Schinke, S. (1978). Teenage pregnancy: The need for multiple casework services. *Social Casework, 59*(7), 406–410.

Schinke, S. P., Blythe, B. J., Gilchrist, & Burt, G. A. (1981). Primary prevention of adolescent pregnancy. *Social Work with Groups, 4*(1,2), 121–135.

Schore, A. (1994). Affect regulation and the origin of the self. The neurobiology of emotional development. Hillsdale, NJ: Lawrence Erlbaum Associates.

Shah, F., & Zelnick, M. (1981). Parent and peer influence on sexual behavior, contraceptive use, and pregnancy experience of young women. *Journal of Marriage and the Family, 43,* 339–348.

Shapiro, J., & Applegate, J. (2000). The neurobiology of affect regulation: Implications for clinical social work. *Clinical Social Work, 28,* 1–28.

Shapiro, J., & Mangelsdorf, S. (1994). The determinants of parenting competence in adolescent mothers. *Journal of Youth and Adolescence, 23*(6), 621–641.

Shapiro, V., Shapiro, J., & Paret, I. (2001). *Complex adoption and assisted reproductive technology: A developmental approach to clinical practice.* New York: The Guilford Press.

Sexuality Information and Education Council of the United States (SIECUS). (2001). Exclusive purpose: Abstinence-only proponents create federal entitlement welfare program. *SIECUS Report Article, 24*(4).

Siegel, D. (1999). *The developing mind: Toward neurobiology of interpersonal experience.* New York: The Guilford Press.

Sims, K., & Luster, T. (2002). Factors related to early subsequent pregnancies and second births among adolescent mothers in a family support program. *Journal of Family Issues, 23*(8), 1006–1031.

Singh, S., & Darroch, J. E. (1999). Trends in sexual activity among adolescent American women: 1982–1995. *Family Planning Perspectives, 31*(5), 212–219.

Smith, D. S., & Hindus, M. S. (1975). Premarital pregnancy in America 1640–1971: An overview and interpretation. *Journal of Interdisciplinary History, 4,* 537–570.

Smith, M. F. (1934). Changing emphasis in case work with unmarried mothers. *The Family, 14,* 310–317.

South Carolina Campaign to Prevent Teen Pregnancy. (2001). *2008 Fact sheet.* Retrieved November 3, 2008, from

Stack, C. (1974). *All our kin.* New York: Harper and Row Pub.

Steele, M., Steel, H., Croft, C., & Fonagy, P. (1999). Infant mother attachment at one year predicts children's understanding of mixed emotions at 6 years. *Social Development, 8,* 161–178.

Steinberg, L. (2003). Is decision making the right framework for research on adolescent risk-taking? In D. Romer (Ed.), *Reducing adolescent risk: Toward an integrated approach* (pp. 18–24). Thousand Oaks, CA: Sage Publications, Inc.

Stern, D. (1985). *The interpersonal world of the infant: A view from psychoanalysis and developmental psychology.* New York: Basic Books.

Stevens, J. W. (1997). African-American female adolescent identity development: A three-dimensional perspective. *Child Welfare, 2,* 145–172.

Stevens-Simon, C., & McAnarney, E.R. (1994). Childhood victimization: Relationships to adolescent pregnancy outcome. *Child Abuse and Neglect, 18*(7), 569–575.

Stock, J. L., Bell, M. A., Boyer, D. K., & Connell, F. A. (1997). Adolescent pregnancy and sexual risk-taking among sexually abused girls. *Family Planning Perspectives, 29*(5), 200–203, 227.

Stouthhamer–Loeber, M., & Wei, E. H. (1998). The precursors of young fatherhood and its effects on delinquency of teenage males. *North American Journal of Psychology, 4*(1), 81–92.

Stream Pictures from Family Records. (1924). The unmarried mother. *The Family, 5,* 228–231.

Sun, S. S., Schubert, C. M., Liang, R., Roche, A. F., Kulin, H. E., Lee, P. A., et al. (2005). Is sexual maturity occurring earlier among U.S. children? *Journal of Adolescent Health, 37*(5):345–55.

Substance Abuse and Mental Health Services Administration. (SAMH-SA) (1999; 2000). National Survey in Drug Use and Health. Available at: http://www.oas.samhsa.gov/NSDUH.

Thomas, E., & Rickel, A. (1995). Teen Pregnancy and Maladjustment: A study of base rates. *Journal of Community Psychology, 23*(3), 200–215.

Thompson, M. P., & Kingree, J. B. (1998). The frequency and impact of violent trauma among pregnant substance abusers. *Addictive Behaviors, 23*(2), 257–262.

Thornberry, T. P., Smith, C. A., & Howard, G. J. (1997). Risk factors for teenage fatherhood. *Journal of Marriage the Family, 59*(3), 505–522.

Toray, T., Coughlin, C., Vuchinich, S., & Patricelli, P. (1991). Gender differences associated with adolescent substance abuse: Comparisons and implications for treatment. Family Relations. *Journal of Applied Family and Child Studies, 40*(3), 338–344.

Trad, P. (1993). Substance abuse in adolescent mothers: Strategies for diagnosis, treatment and prevention. *Journal of Substance Abuse Treatment, 10,* 421–431.

Trenholm,C., Devaney, B., Fortson, K., Clark, M, Quay, L., & Wheeler, J. (2008). Impacts of abstinence education on teen sexual activity, risk of pregnancy, and risk of sexually transmitted diseases. *Journal of Policy Analysis and Management, 27*(2), 255–276.

U C ANR Latina/o Teen Pregnancy Prevention Workgroup. (2004). *Best Practices in Teen Pregnancy Prevention Handbook* (2nd ed.). Oakland, CA: University of California Cooperative Extension.

U.S. Department of Health and Human Services. (2000). *A national strategy to prevent teen pregnancy: Annual report 1999–2000.* Washington, DC: Assistant Secretary for Planning and Evaluation.

Unger, J. B., Molina, G. B., & Teran, L. (2000). Perceived consequences of teenage childbearing among adolescent girls in an urban sample. *Journal of Adolescent Health, 26,* 205–212.

Upchurch, D. M., Aneshensel, C. S., Sucoff, C. A., & Levy-Storms, L. (1999). Neighborhood and family contexts of sexual activity. *Journal of Marriage and the Family, 61,* 920–933.

Uziel–Miller, N. D., & Lyons, J. S. (2000). Specialized substance abuse treatment for women and their children: An analysis of program design. *Journal of Substance Abuse Treatment, 19*(4), 355–367.

Van Wormer, K. S. (1995). *Alcoholism treatment: A social work perspective.* Chicago: Nelson–Hall Publishers.

Veach T.L., Sheld, H., Pistorello, J., Arkowitz, L. and Chappel, J.N. (1995). Perinatal substance use patterns in obstetrics-gynecology. Substance Abuse, Vol 16(2), Jun 1995. pp. 115–123.

Ventura, S. J. (1997). Recent trends and variations in nonmarital childbearing. *Children Today, 24*(2), 12–13.

Ventura, S. J., Curtin, S. C., & Mathews, T. J. (2000). Variations in teenage birth rates, 1991–1998: National and state trends. National Vital Statistics Reports, 48. Hyattsville, MD: National Center for Health Statistics.

Ventura, S. J., Mosher, W. D., Curtin, C. S., Abma, J. C., & Henshaw, S. (2000). Trends in pregnancies and pregnancy rates by outcome: Estimates for the United States, 1976–1996. National Center for Health Statistics. *Vital Health Statistics, 21*.

Ventura, S. J., Abma, J. C., Mosher, W. D., & Henshaw, S. K. (2008). *Estimated pregnancy rates by outcome for the United States, 1990–2004*. National Vital Statistics Reports. (Vol 56, no.15). Hyattsville, MD: National Center for Health Statistics.

Veroff, J., Kulka, R., & Douvan, E. (1981). *Mental health in America: Patterns of help-seeking form 1957 to 1976*. New York: Basic Books.

Vincent, C. (1961). *Unmarried mothers*. New York: Free Press of Glencoe.

Vinovskis, M. A. (1988). An "epidemic" of adolescent pregnancy? Some historical and policy considerations. New York: Oxford University Press.

Walling, A. D. (2001). Marijuana use during pregnancy. *American Family Physician, 63*(12), 2463.

Ward, M., Botyanski, N., Plunkett, S., & Carlson, E. (1991). *The concurrent and predictive validity of the AAI for adolescent mothers*. Paper presented at the biennial meeting of the Society for Research in Child Development, Seattle, WA.

Watts, G. F., & Nagy, S. (2000). Sociodemographic factors, attitudes, and expectations toward adolescent coitus. *American Journal of Health Behavior, 24*(4): 309–317. Retrieved September 23, 2008, from waysandmeans. house.gov/media/pdf/greenbook2003/AppendixM.pdf.

Weisman, C. S., Plichta, S., Nathanson, C. A., Chase, G. A., Ensminger, M., E., & Robinson, J. C. (1991). Adolescent women's contraceptive decision making. *Journal of Health and Social Behavior, 32*(2), 130–144.

Whitaker, D. J., Miller, K. S., & Clark, L. F. (2000). Reconceptualizing adolescent sexual behavior: Beyond did they or didn't they? *Family Planning Perspectives, 32*(3), 111–117.

Whitaker, D. J., & Miller, K. S., (2000). Parent–adolescent discussions about sex and condoms: Impact of peer influences of sexual risk behavior. *Journal of Adolescent Research, 15*(2), 251–273.

Whitbeck, L., Yoder, K. A., Hoyt, D. R., & Conger, R. D. (1999). Early adolescent sexual activity: A developmental study. *Journal of Marriage and the Family, 61*, 934–946.

Whitman, T., Borkowski, J., Schellenbach, C., & Nath, P. (1987). Predicting and understanding developmental delay of children of adolescent mothers: A multidimensional approach. *American Journal of Mental Deficiency, 92*, 40–56.

Widmer, E. D. (1997). Influence of older siblings on the initiation sexual intercourse. *Journal of Marriage and the Family, 59*, 928–938.

Wilson, B. & Miller, R. (2003). Examining strategies for culturally grounded prevention: A review. *AIDS Education and Prevention, 15*, 184–220.

Wilson, K., Goodson, B., Pruitt., Buhi, E., & Davis–Gunnels, E. (2005). A review of 21 curricula for abstinence-only-until-marriage programs. *Journal of School Health, 75*(3), 90–98.

Winnicott, D. W. (1965). *The maturational processes and the facilitating environment: Studies in the theory of emotional development*. Madison, WI: International Universities Press.

Wisconsin Division of Child and Family Services. (n.d.) *Brighter futures initiative*. Retrieved October 9, 2008, from http://dhs.wisconsin.gov/sca2008/PDF/BFI.pdf.

Witkin, S. L., & Harrison, W. D. (2001). Whose evidence and for what purpose? *Social Work, 46*(4), 293–296.

Witte, K. (1997). Preventing teen pregnancy through persuasive communications: realities, myths and the hard-fact truths. *Journal of Community Health, 22*(2), 137–154.

Wu, T., Mendola, P., & Buck, G. M. (2002). Ethnic differences in the presence of secondary sex characteristics and menarche among U.S. girls: The Third national health and nutrition examination. *Pediatrics, 110*(4):752–757.

Xie, H., Cairns, B.D., & Cairns, R.B. (2001). Predicting teen motherhood and teen fatherhood: Individual characteristics and peer affiliations. *Social Development, 10*(4), 488–509.

Young, L. (1947). The unmarried mother's decision about her baby. *Journal of Social Casework, 28*, 27–34.

Young, L. (1954). *Out of wedlock*. New York: McGraw Hill, Co.

Zabin, L. S., & Hayward, S. C. (1993). *Adolescent sexual behavior and childbearing*. Newbury Park: Sage Publications.

Zanis, D. (2005). Use of a sexual abstinence only curriculum with sexually active youths. *Social Work, 27*(1), 59–63.

Zelnick, M., & Kantner, J. (1977). Sexual and contraceptive experiences of young women in the United States, 1971–1976. *Family Planning Perspectives, (March-April)*, 55–73.

Zelnick, M., Kantner, J. F., & Ford, K. (1981). *Sex and pregnancy in adolescence*. Beverly Hills, CA: Sage.

INDEX